How Can Nurses Survive Bullying Environments?

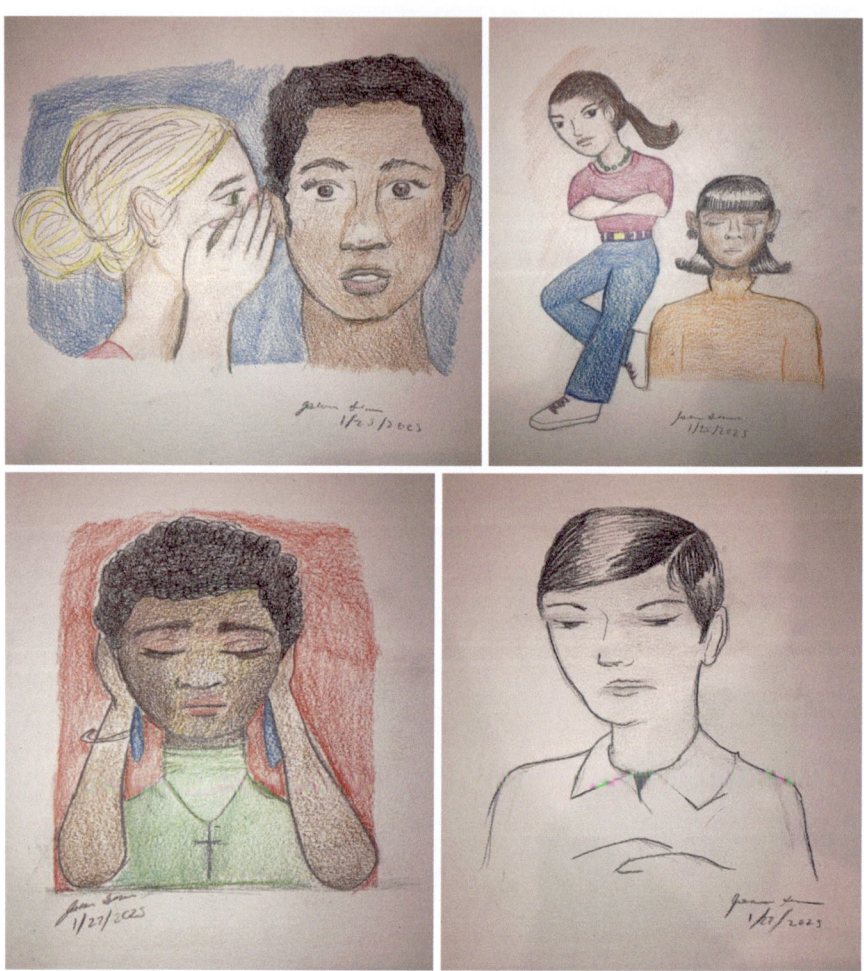

Bullying is a distortion, a fallacy in reality. No one has power over you unless you give your power to them. You feel broken, naked, and exposed. But there is a light that provides peace, strength, and hope. The truth is revealed. Lies exposed, and you emerge stronger than you were before.
Illustrations by Joshua Green

Cheryl Green

How Can Nurses Survive Bullying Environments?

The Hollow Theory

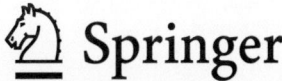

Cheryl Green
Abilene Christian University
Abilene, TX, USA

ISBN 978-3-031-86616-6   ISBN 978-3-031-86617-3 (eBook)
https://doi.org/10.1007/978-3-031-86617-3

© The Editor(s) (if applicable) and The Author(s), under exclusive license to Springer Nature Switzerland AG 2025

This work is subject to copyright. All rights are solely and exclusively licensed by the Publisher, whether the whole or part of the material is concerned, specifically the rights of translation, reprinting, reuse of illustrations, recitation, broadcasting, reproduction on microfilms or in any other physical way, and transmission or information storage and retrieval, electronic adaptation, computer software, or by similar or dissimilar methodology now known or hereafter developed.
The use of general descriptive names, registered names, trademarks, service marks, etc. in this publication does not imply, even in the absence of a specific statement, that such names are exempt from the relevant protective laws and regulations and therefore free for general use.
The publisher, the authors and the editors are safe to assume that the advice and information in this book are believed to be true and accurate at the date of publication. Neither the publisher nor the authors or the editors give a warranty, expressed or implied, with respect to the material contained herein or for any errors or omissions that may have been made. The publisher remains neutral with regard to jurisdictional claims in published maps and institutional affiliations.

This Springer imprint is published by the registered company Springer Nature Switzerland AG
The registered company address is: Gewerbestrasse 11, 6330 Cham, Switzerland

If disposing of this product, please recycle the paper.

This book is dedicated to those nurses and non-nurses who have experienced bullying in the workplace. You will heal and you will survive. You will grow stronger as you realize that the bully or bullies are but a small whisper, a speck of dust blowing aimlessly in the wind. Take your vision and dreams back, you are radiantly priceless!

Preface

The Hollow Theory was developed in 2018 by Dr. Cheryl Green, a licensed clinical social worker, registered nurse, and educator, after witnessing the mental and physical deterioration of nurses in the workplace by their fellow nurses who targeted them for the act of bullying. The nurses shared their bullying experiences with Dr. Green, detailing how the bully or bullies began to display derogatory behaviors toward them. These derogatory behaviors consisted of lying and fabricating stories regarding the nurse's work performance, belittling them in front of colleagues as if they were of sub-intelligence, sabotaging their work, blaming, and mobbing behaviors where a group of nurses were involved in attempting to bring harm to the targeted nurse's character.

For nurses who experience The Hollow, they begin to withdraw, become depressed, and seemingly, perseverate on the bullying behaviors. Psychologically, untreated, these nurses can develop anxiety and/or panic disorders or depression. Some individuals can actually become suicidal as they begin to feel hopeless and helpless in their situation. Physical symptoms such as gastrointestinal problems, headaches, and hypertension can develop because of nurses' consistent exposure to the stress of the bullying situation.

Healthy workplaces must be advocated for by nurses and their employers to ensure that bullying is not tolerated and the lives of nurses are valued and respected. The Hollow Theory is not only a theory to recognize and support bullied nurses, but to advocate for and support every employee that has or is experiencing workplace bullying.

Abilene, TX, USA   Cheryl Green

Contents

1	**Dysfunction Within a Profession of Caritas**	1
	Introduction	1
	Therapeutic Communication	1
	Dysfunction	1
	A Systemic Problem	1
	Bullying Manifestation	2
	Direct Harm	2
	Indirect Harm	2
	Nurse Suicide	3
	Lamenting	4
	Wilderness Stories	5
	Questions to Contemplate: Let's Get to Work!	7
	References	8
2	**Origins of The Hollow**	11
	Introduction	11
	Bullying Characteristics	11
	Bullying Target Types	12
	Personal Losses Endured by Bullied Persons	12
	What Is The Hollow Theory?	13
	Survival Unimagined	13
	Organizational Impact of Bullying	14
	Cold Communications	15
	Activity: Poof!	16
	Meditation for Contemplation	16
	References	17
3	**Structured Workplace Chaos**	19
	Introduction	19
	Hypothetical Case Study: "That Is Not True!"	20
	Groupthink	20
	Territorialism	21
	Sabotage	21
	The Depleted Nurse	21
	Can't Do It	22

Structural Chaos in the Workplace ... 22
Structural Empowerment ... 22
Incivility ... 23
Summary ... 23
Examples of Structured Workplace Chaos ... 24
Activity: Identification of Bully Roles and Hidden Agendas in the Workplace Environment ... 24
    Workplace Scenarios ... 24
Activities Acknowledging Workplace Ingenuity ... 28
    Recognizing Healthy and Not So Healthy Workplace Communication Responses ... 28
Answers ... 29
    Recognizing Healthy and Not So Healthy Workplace Communication Responses ... 29
Activity ... 30
    Identification of Mindsets ... 30
References ... 31

4 Patients Matter ... 33
Introduction ... 33
Patients ... 33
Healthcare Organizations ... 34
Patient-Centered Healthcare ... 34
The Assumption of Sick Role ... 35
Nurses and Patients ... 35
Forms of Communication ... 36
Interpersonal Theory ... 37
    The Value of Effective Communication ... 37
    The Angry Patient ... 37
Summary ... 38
References ... 38

5 Unprovoked ... 41
Unprovoked ... 41
Harming Others ... 42
The Bewilderment of Gaslighting ... 42
Dominance ... 43
Narcissistic Personality Disorder 301.81 (F60.81) ... 43
Gaslighting in the Workplace ... 43
Heal Thyself ... 44
Moving Forward ... 44
Summary ... 45
Activity ... 45
    Adult Drawing for Healing and Clarity of Situation ... 45
Activity ... 47
    The Act of Moving Forward ... 47
References ... 48

6	**Shallow**	49
	Shallow	49
	Treading Water	49
	Difficult Conversations	50
	Hidden Conflict	50
	The Maintenance of Truth	51
	Overexposed	51
	Not an Option	52
	The Workplace	52
	Exit, Voice, Loyalty, and Neglect	52
	Summary: No Depth	53
	Activity	53
	Activity	55
	Depth or No Depth: Shallow	55
	References	55
7	**The Depths of Forgetfulness**	57
	Forgetfulness	57
	Forgiveness	58
	The Danger of Workplace Bullying	59
	Quiet Quitting	59
	Wronged	60
	Summary: Unearthing Forgetfulness	60
	Putting Forgiveness into Practice	61
	A Personal Activity	61
	References	62
8	**The Depths of Regret**	65
	Regret Defined	65
	The Hollow	65
	The Targets	66
	The Broken Bully	66
	Scenario 1: Bully Overreaction	67
	The Emotional Voice	67
	Regret in the Workplace: Why Is This Unhealthy Behavior Tolerated Anyway	68
	Navigating Workplace Change in Real Time	69
	Activity	70
	Change	70
	A Contemplation Activity	73
	Regret	73
	References	74
9	**Simplifying Life**	75
	Work-Life Balance	75
	Simplifying Life	76
	Here Is an Idea: Just Go to the Workplace to Work	77
	Why Do I Suffer at Work?	77

	Workplace Norms	78
	Who Says "No" Is Such a Bad Word in the Workplace?	78
	Common Sense	79
	And So, I Recall: Learning from the Past	79
	References	81
10	**A Coverage of Eyes and Ears**	**83**
	Eyes and Ears	83
	Secondary Trauma	83
	Summary	84
	References	84
11	**Is a State of Calm Achievable?**	**85**
	A History of Abuse	85
	Calm	85
	Achievable	86
	Activity	86
	The Use of Mindfulness in Healing from The Hollow	86
	Counseling	88
	References	89
12	**Arise and Journey More**	**91**
	Arise	91
	Journey More	91
	Emotional Support	92
	Personal Growth	92
	Empowerment	93
	References	94

Conclusion: The Gratitude Effect Booklet 97

About the Author

Cheryl Green PhD, DNP, RN, LCSW, CNL, CNE, MAC, FAPA. The beauty of living is the experience of pain, happiness, sorrow, and life disruptions. No one is excluded from hardship in life. When bullied, human being-to-human being, the unconscionable occurs, both emotionally and physically, the body is impacted, suffering spiritual, physical, and mental harm. The latter can be prevented, when the person or persons who are being bullied view the very act of bullying for what it is, the fear and insecurities of the bully or bullies. Cheryl Green is happily married to William with two adult children. She believes in the resiliency of others and that change can occur at any stage in life—the negative changed to the positive.

Dysfunction Within a Profession of Caritas

Introduction

Caritas subjectively, is the individual's personal drive to provide and exhibit care to others. The care exhibited by the individual can be emotional, physical, and spiritual in nature. The Theory of Human Caring was developed by Jean Watson (2008). The Theory of Human Caring is a framework for the delivery of nursing care to patients that focuses upon the nurse-patient therapeutic relationship (Watson, 2009). The nurse in the role of a caring and compassionate healthcare professional uses this healing relationship to promote caritas during a time in life when patients/clients are most vulnerable, either physiologically or psychologically.

Therapeutic Communication

Dysfunction

The premise of **dysfunction** is the absence of order. Chaos is a distractor. Amidst noise, subtle complaints, frustrations, and anger, persons acting as *disruptors* within the work environment seek to lie and undermine their fellow workers, often without provocation. Compartmentally, units, departments, schools, and other organizationally defined teams can either thrive, survive, or slowly disintegrate under the weight of denigration perpetuated by persons or a person who bullies.

A Systemic Problem

According to Edmonson and Zelonka (2019), bullying behaviors have been found to exist before nursing school and persist throughout a nurse's careers. Nurse bullying quickly becomes a systematic problem because financially, organizations are impacted. Patient satisfaction scores are lower (Hospital Consumer Assessment of Healthcare Providers and Systems [HCAPS]) because patients are treated within environments of high nursing stress whereby there may be a higher likelihood of nursing errors, and there is a pattern of nursing turnover. Hence, each time a nurse leaves their position related to bullying, the bottom-line costs for hospitals are impacted. While bullied nurses can be any age, turnover is seen more often within nurses in their first job which is often that of a bedside nurse.

Turnover of bedside nurses is of particular concern. The current estimated cost of a nurse leaving the bedside increased by 20.7% and is $56,300.00 per nurse. Statistically, on average, hospitals within the United States are losing $3.9 to $5.8 million dollars annually (Nursing Solutions Inc., 2024). If hospitals are able to significantly decrease their nurse turnover, a savings/cost of $262,500 annually could be obtained. Given that it can take 3 months or more to recruit nurses with clinical practice experience, the vacancy for registered nurses is nationally 9.9% and the RN Recruitment Difficulty Index averages a total of 86 days (Nursing Solutions Inc., 2024).

Bullying Manifestation

Manifestations of bullying behaviors can be subtle or direct. For example, a bully may lie, attempt to discredit someone through distorting what they say or do, or spread rumors. Other bullying can be based on identity-based hate (e.g., racism, religion, gender, etc.). Bullies may overtly yell at, ignore, or embarrass the person they are targeting as a means to gain power over them. Remember, bullies are often very insecure and fearful of coworkers that are more knowledgeable than themselves, happy, or accomplished in their specialty areas.

Direct Harm

Direct harm in bullying tends to be openly done in the presence of others, openly humiliating someone with their co-workers being present, silencing or pretending the targeted person did not say anything. Hostile and antagonistic body language, blaming and shaming, yelling, punching and pushing, emailing, texting, or writing angry messages are behaviors that are more direct. With direct harm, the bully has reached the point of comfort. Hence the bully's behavior has gone unchecked or corrected by the organization, so the bully or bullies openly express their dislike of their target(s) without retribution (Praslova et al., 2022).

Indirect Harm

When a person is indirectly harmed during bullying, persons may experience less than adequate transfer of information from colleagues in order to perform their jobs;

shared information with vital gaps, hence, occurs, with the goal of sabotaging. Bullied persons can also experience circumvention of information and spreading of rumors (Edmonson & Zelonka, 2019; Praslova et al., 2022). Ultimately, the bully or bullies are focused upon the failure of the affected person in their ability to do and successfully complete their work. Within the workplace, an employer that is intuitively tracking these behaviors after an initial incident should involve a human resource representative to investigate all future events to rule out patterns of lying and sabotage. However, in absence of actual disciplinary action of the bully or bullies, once patterns have been identified, behaviors will continue. The affected nurse, if resilient, can with ease, address what they know to be false information. However, not all nurses are comfortable in doing so, and hence, affected nurses may begin to feel helpless and hopeless within the situation.

Nurse Suicide

Historically, the profession of nursing has been wrought with staff division, emotionally embattled nurses, and physically ill nurses because of a long-standing bullying problem within the profession. Suicides committed by nurses who hurt (Davis et al., 2021; Lee & Friese, 2021; Stephenson, 2018) have occurred within the context of nurses being bullied by fellow nurses in the workplace and the day-to-day stress of delivering healthcare to patients in a fast-paced environment. Davidson et al. (2018) in a discussion paper to raise awareness about the problem of **nurse suicides** for the National Academies of Medicine shared that there had been minimal tracking of nurse suicides and organizational responses to help nurses in comparison to physicians and other professions (e.g., police officers, educators, firefighters, and military personnel). Davidson et al. (2018) noted that compassion and caring can take a toll on nurses. Ethical issues at work, lateral violence, staffing shortages, moral distress (nurse is prevented from doing what the nurse knows is right to do), blame, medical and medication errors, near misses and omissions in the care of patients/clients, and inappropriate treatment are just a few examples of what practicing nurses must deal with while delivering healthcare. Collective risk factors for nurse suicide include the knowledge of how to use toxic substances and lethal doses of medications, personal and work-related stressors, smoking, depression and undertreatment of depression, and substance abuse (Davidson et al., 2018; Lee & Friese, 2021).

Between the years 2017 and 2018, it is estimated that 729 nurses within the United States ended their lives by suicide (Davis et al., 2021). According to the National Academy of Sciences, Engineering, and Medicine (2019), burnout of healthcare clinicians threatens the quality of patient care delivered. Hence it is imperative that health systems' organizational leadership act to address their workers' stress. Limited human resources, equitable workload challenges, improvement in documentation and administrative processes, and assignment of non-nursing duties to nursing staff must be readily addressed. The National Academy of Sciences, Engineering, and Medicine (2019) recommends that healthcare organizations and systems senior leadership be held accountable for nurses' safety and partner with nurses to create healthier work environments. Other recommendations to address nurse suicide include the American Rescue Plan Act of 2021 (Congress.gov, 2021–2022) that has allotted monies to promote mental healthcare for healthcare professionals, implementation of the Healer Education Assessment and Referral (HEAR) suicide prevention program in some organizations (Davidson et al., 2018), emphasis on self-care (Zhang et al., 2020), and the potential implementation of a socio-ecological framework to decrease nurse suicides at a societal level through policy development, changes in the working environment, and practice changes (Wasserman et al., 2020).

Lamenting

To **lament** is to experience a deep sadness over an event that occurred in one's life. The death of spouse or child or the loss of something or someone of great significance in one's life can cause sorrow, grief, and regret. When nurses experience The Hollow, bewilderment as to why the bullying or gaslighting is occurring to them can be a precipitant to their lamenting. As the mind recalls story after story of situations whereby bullying or gaslighting was the theme of conversational content or physical actions directed toward them, nurses begin to feel anxious. Their overwhelming anxiety disturbingly leading to feelings of hopelessness and helplessness as they mentally fight to differentiate what they perceive versus what is actually happening to them.

Lamenting actually occurs as a result of the recall of times of peace and happiness in the workplace that is remembered by the affected nurse. The bewilderment, the affected nurse asking themselves, "How and why is this occurring? Why is this happening to me?" Shrouded by either an environment that either supports the nurse(s) with their bullying situation or a workplace that decidedly ignores bullying, choosing to view the nurse or nurses' situation as an individual problem only and not potentially an organizational issue, The Hollow will either continue to grow or be intervened upon and ended abruptly. Whatever the organization's decision, human lives are impacted both on the part of the nurse and the patients that the lamenting nurse provides care to as he or she is experiencing workplace bullying. Distracted, unfulfilled, anxious, fearful, worried, and scattered in their ability to thoroughly exercise clinical judgment and critical thinking, nurses affected by The Hollow, although historically good nurses, may not perform well in their delivery of healthcare to the public (Praslova et al., 2022; NSI, 2018, 2023, 2024).

The healthy side of lamenting is its necessity. Human beings must have periods of grief and sorrow in order to process life events. In absence of the ability to process a harm that is mental, physical, or spiritual, persons are left vulnerable because they are unable to protect themselves from the event occurring again in their lives. Lamenting provides a life lesson. The life lesson of lamenting is that a person or persons can survive difficult situations and do well in their lives. Losses experienced through The Hollow can include self-esteem, insecurity with one's previously mastered skills, self-hatred, and a general feeling of awkwardness and not belonging. Unfortunately, the latter feelings not only manifest themselves in the workplace environment of origination but also impact the private life of the nurse or nurses affected, hence the risk for the development of mental illness (e.g., depression, anxiety, etc.) and physical illness. Of even more concern, the nurse may have accompanied sleep deprivation, decrease or increase in appetite, and a decrease in the ability to concentrate. Physical and mental vulnerabilities can also increase the potential for the development of suicidal ideation and lead to an actual suicide attempt (Halter, 2022).

The result of successful lamenting is the realization that life is filled with imperfection and that we ourselves are imperfect. Because we must daily interact with imperfection, we must learn to be kind to ourselves in every situation. Being kind to ourselves gives us permission to recognize and act on the correction of the negative behaviors of others toward us. We do not have to tolerate the dysfunction of other people in our lives, nor do others have to tolerate our negative behaviors in their lives.

Wilderness Stories

Directions Wilderness stories are stories told by nurses that have experienced bullying and share how it has impacted their lives. Please read each of the ten short stories and discuss with another person or within a group of peers how each situation may have impacted the lives of the affected nurses. These are hypothetical stories written for the purpose of educating others about the short-term and long-term effects of bullying:

1. I could not believe that she thought it was o.k. to yell at me at a staff meeting. My boss said absolutely nothing. It is as if the yelling episode never happened. I cannot understand how being inappropriate in a professional work environment is tolerated.
2. I am done with being treated like an ignorant child by my preceptor. My preceptor and I have met four times with the manager. The first time we met with the manager, it was 2 weeks into my 8-week orientation. My preceptor shared with a patient's wife that she had to watch everything I did to ensure I did not make an error and "kill someone." I have been a nurse for 10 years. What a ridiculous and extremely rude thing to say. I am done with my preceptor and this place!
3. Who would have thought I would be bullied by a 22-year-old with less than 1 year of clinical nursing experience? I am 62 years old and I have a "kid" lying and trying to set me up. Trying to explain this nonsense to a Human Resource representative is even more hilarious. No support, absolutely no support.
4. We do not know quite how to react when we observe Mike get teased and belittled by our director. Mike is a really nice guy and a hard worker. I just do not understand why our director is unnecessarily hard on him. Should we come to Mike's defense? He is starting to look very depressed and tired of the director's behavior.

5. I vomit before and after I have to deal with them. They are like wolves, travelling in a pack. No one takes responsibility for the acknowledgement of the negative behaviors the three of these women bring to the workplace. I don't know how much longer I will be at this place. And to think, I planned to advance my career and, eventually, retire from this job.
6. Craig is so comfortable lying. It is as if his defamation of other's character and stealing of their ideas bring no regret nor discomfort to his consciousness. How can persons affected pretend no damage has been done. How do people sell their own souls and identity to stay in the good graces of a person that has absolutely no respect for them?
7. Lately, I have been having thoughts of just ending it all. I just cannot take being bullied anymore at work. I am depressed and feel hopeless and helpless.
8. I feel paranoid sometimes. Being gaslighted was tough. I just do not trust people and I am not sure if I ever will. Should I see a therapist or counselor? I am not sure how to move forward.
9. My stomach hurts and I have a headache. I have always put a job…a career before family and everything else. When you go through harassment in the workplace for nothing you personally did, you question who you are and who you abandoned for a job. Family, friends, a husband, a child…all of these are priceless. To think, I put a job before all that mattered most. The harassment I experienced on the job is proof that a job is never important than those you love.
10. Pushed and shoved in silence. A smirk and then laughter. Belittled in front of others. I am much more than how a bully perceives me. I am loved by others and valued. I will move on and be just fine.

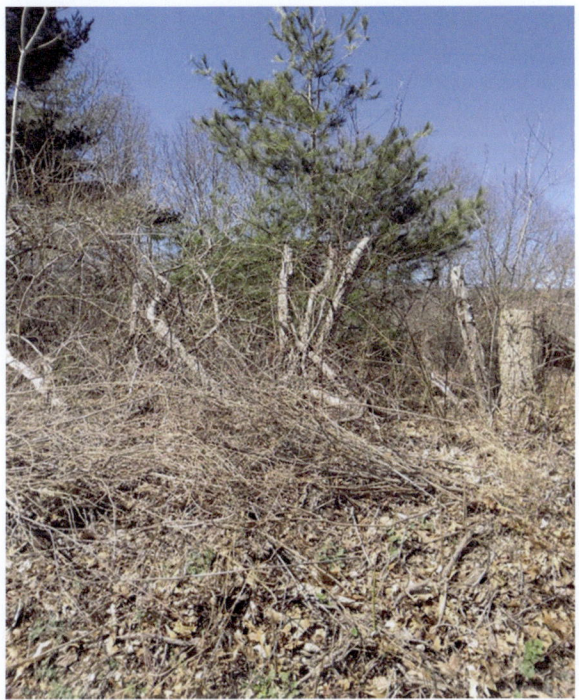

Brush in Spring Time

Questions to Contemplate: Let's Get to Work!

Directions Read and discuss the following questions about dysfunction within the profession of nursing. Consider what you can do to help improve work environments for nurses. Contemplate immediate reparative responses that can be made by nurses, professional organizations, and the healthcare systems and organizations which employee nurses:

1. Why would a profession based on caritas be so stressful?
2. How early should nurse bullying be intervened upon?
3. Is there a pattern of bullying within the nursing profession?
4. Can nurses be given support earlier by their organizations with bullying prevention?
5. Should nursing leadership be held responsible for knowingly allowing bullying to occur in the workplace?
6. Should human resources be held accountable if consistent patterns of bullying on a particular clinical unit or other healthcare workplace setting are permitted or not addressed directly at all?

7. Is it possible for nurses to be insulated from factors contributing to nurse suicide?
8. What other actions could be taken to address nurse suicide?
9. Is nurse suicide a public health issue?
10. What does it mean to the nursing profession to experience another nursing death by suicide? What are the implications?

References

American Rescue Plan Act of 2021, Pub. L. No. H.R. 1319. (2021). *Congress.gov.* https://www.congress.gov/bill/117th-congress/house-bill/1319/text

Davis, M. A., Cher, B. A. Y, Friese, C. R., Bynum, J. P. W. (2021). Association of US nurse and physician occupation with risk of suicide. *JAMA Psychiatry, 78*(6):651–658. https://doi.org/10.1001/jamapsychiatry.2021.0154

Davidson, J., Mendis, J., Stuck, A. R., DeMichele, G., & Zisook, S. (2018). *Nurse suicide: Breaking the silence.* National Academy of Medicine. https://nam.edu/nurse-suicide-breaking-the-silence/

Edmonson, C., & Zelonka, C. (2019). Our own worst enemies. The nurse bullying academic. *Nursing Administration Quarterly, 43*(3), 274–279. https://journals.lww.com/naqjournal/fulltext/2019/07000/our_own_worst_enemies__the_nurse_bullying_epidemic.12.aspx

Halter, M. J. (2022). *Varcarolis' foundations of psychiatric-mental health nursing: A clinical approach* (9th ed.). Elsevier.

Lee, K. A., & Friese, C. R. (2021). Deaths by suicide among nurses: A rapid response call. *Journal of Psychosocial Nursing and Mental Health Services, 59*(8), 3–4. https://doi.org/10.3928/02793695-20210625-01

National Academy of Sciences Engineering and Medicine. (2019). *Taking-action against clinician burnout: A systems approach to professional Well-being.* The National Academies Press. https://doi.org/10.17226/25521

Nursing Solutions Inc. (2018). *2018 National health care retention & RN staffing report.* http://www.nsinursingsolutions.com/files/assets/library/retention-institute/nationalhealthcarernretentionreport2018.pdf

Nursing Solutions Inc. (2023). *2023 National health care retention & RN staffing report.* https://www.nsinursingsolutions.com/Documents/Library/NSI_National_Health_Care_Retention_Report.pdf

Nursing Solutions Inc. (2024). *2024 NSI national health care retention & RN Staffing Report.* https://www.nsinursingsolutions.com/documents/library/nsi_national_health_care_retention_report.pdf

Praslova, L. N., Carucci, R., & Stokes, C. (2022). How bullying manifests at work—And how to stop it. *Harvard Business Review.* https://hbr.org/2022/11/how-bullying-manifests-at-work-and-how-to-stop-it

Stephenson, J. (2018). Nursing director to meet family of nurse who said she was bullied before taking own life. *Nursing Times, 114*(8), 131. ISSN: 0954-7762.

Wasserman, D., Iosue, M., Wuestefeld, A., & Carli, V. (2020). Adaptation of evidence-based suicide prevention strategies during and after the COVID-19 pandemic. *World Psychiatry: Official Journal of the World Psychiatric Association, 19*(3), 294–306. https://doi.org/10.1002/wps.20801

Watson, J. (2008). Nursing the philosophy and science of caring (Revised ed.). University Press of Colorado.

References

Watson, J. (2009, Spring). Caring science and human caring theory: Transforming personal and professional practices of nursing and healthcare. *Journal of Health and Human Services Administration, 31*, 466–482. https://pubmed.ncbi.nlm.nih.gov/19385422/

Zhang, X.-J., Song, Y., Jiang, T., Ding, N., & Shi, T.-Y. (2020). Interventions to reduce burnout of physicians and nurses: An overview of systematic reviews and meta-analyses. *Medicine, 99*(26), e20992. https://doi.org/10.1097/MD.0000000000020992

Origins of The Hollow

2

Learning Objectives

1. Explain The Hollow Theory and the physical and emotional manifestations within nurses affected by workplace bullying.
2. Describe the potential for physiological and psychological decline of the nurse affected by sustained bullying in the workplace.
3. Decipher ways in which nurses affected by The Hollow can successfully recover with support.

Introduction

Bullying Characteristics

Bullying is the action(s) taken by a person or group of people toward another person(s) with the intent of producing physical or emotional harm. In the study of different ways that nurses bully one another, the literature identifies behaviors such as cyberbullying (Park & Choi, 2019), with bullying occurring on Internet platforms. Additionally, nurse-to-nurse bullying can consist of mobbing (groups of individuals who are jealous of another person's skill level in the workplace bully and attempt to intimidate the person; Valclavikova & Kozakova, 2022), rudeness, lying, gossip, singling out (not being invited to work events fellow employees are all participating within), attempting to attack one's character, name-calling, sabotaging of another's work, and joy-stealing (Heinrich, 2007).

Rude Boy, Rude Girl

In the West Indian culture, a "rude boy or rude girl" was someone within the subculture that was involved in gangster activities or spent time on street corners attempting to make a living, as they were unable to secure work. The rude boy and rude girl were usually unemployed and had difficulty surviving because of their financial and social isolation. Historically, the terms rude boy and rude girl originated in shanty towns within the West Indies. Shanty towns are lower-income areas on the island (The Guardian, 2014; Underground, 2021).

Changes in cultures arise in difficult life situations. In organizations, organizational cultures can shift with changes in employees that bring either negative or positive behaviors to the workplace based upon their own life experiences. Rude boys and rude girls were in fact poor persons who had difficulty finding employment during the 1960s. However, with pride intact, they dressed nicely and moved in the music scene but yet maintained a gangster element.

With regard to "The Hollow," the bully or bullies inflate their own value due to their own insecurities that they make a distinct point of hiding from others. Instead, the bully or bullies project their own frustrations with themselves and their life situations on others. Like the rude boy or rude girl, the bully emerges from complicated life circumstances but makes the wrong decisions in how they view and interact with others who they interact with in "their world" (the world of the bully).

Bullying Target Types

There are approximately four bullying target types. The bullying target types include *downward, horizontal, upward, and mixed*. Downward bullying involves persons in organizational leadership positions whereby they directly supervise and have employees to whom they provide oversight of their work. Bullying that occurs horizontally is lateral, and typically involves coworkers or peers. Upward bullying within the workplace involves subordinates, while mixed bullying usually consists of a workplace clique comprised of subordinates and supervisors. With mixed bullying, the bully or bullies approach their targets directionally, using any of the targeting types of bullying (Praslova et al., 2022).

Personal Losses Endured by Bullied Persons

The losses that persons affected by bully endure can be devastating to their mental and physical health. All areas of their lives are affected. Psychologically, persons may experience posttraumatic stress disorder (PTSD), loss of confidence, nightmares, anxiety, suicidal ideation, insomnia, and depression. Persons may experience a decline in their physical health and have several different physiological problems such as gastrointestinal issues, palpitations, or severe headaches. Additionally, persons with physical health changes may experience burnout and disability with worsening illnesses associated with stress such as an elevated blood pressure or the overuse of drugs or alcohol to self-medicate their trauma (Green, 2019; Praslova et al., 2022).

Socially, persons affected by bullying may lose their professional networks as bullies lie and attempt to attack their character. Friendships are impacted and some persons may experience a loss in their reputation. The person affected by bullying may decide to leave their job, and income or promotion may be given up in order to maintain physical and mental health (Green, 2019; Praslova et al., 2022).

What Is The Hollow Theory?

The **Hollow Theory** is the manifestation of emotional and physical symptomatology related to stress that nurses encounter in workplace settings whereby bullying and incivility are permitted to flourish unabated. Feelings associated with The Hollow include sadness, embittered, feeling hurt, and misunderstood by others. Additionally, affected persons perseverate on incidences of negative behaviors experienced by them from the perpetrator of the act(s) of bullying. Sustained, persons experiencing The Hollow can become physically and mentally ill. Lack of energy, focus, and enthusiasm emerge as part of the perseveration component of The Hollow, whereby affected persons play and replay incidences of bullying. For nurses, and other affected persons, the replaying of incidences of bullying in their minds makes them feel vulnerable, frustrated, and anxious. Accompanied by intermittent tearfulness, productivity in the workplace can ultimately be impacted (Green, 2019; Green, 2020).

Nursing Profession
Nursing is a profession whereby the ability to think analytically, think critically, and exercise clinical judgment in the care of acute and chronically ill patients is a daily expectation. For nurses who experience The Hollow, their ability to concentrate can be affected. Hence, patient safety and the quality in the delivery of nursing care may be compromised.

Nurses that are impacted by The Hollow may make the decision to seek mediation from a nurse manager or a Human Resources representative. Counseling support can be beneficial in helping nurses cope with their anxiety, worry, and perseveration on recalled events of bullying. Counseling can be accessed through the Employee Assistance Program (EAP) through their employer or nurses may seek a private therapist. Licensed mental health professionals can be helpful in helping affected nurses process their bullying experience and maintain their emotional health as affected nurses decide on their next actions in dealing with their unhealthy work situation.

Survival Unimagined

According to the Workplace Bullying Institute, in the United States, 79.3 million employees report being affected by bullying in the workplace (WBI, 2021). Remote workers experience bullying at the rate of 43%; sources of remote workers' bullying include 9% email and 50% via online meetings. Employees are not immune to workplace bullying within leadership positions. Nonmanagement employees who are bullied in the workplace represent 52%, while 40% of managers are bullied, with 30% of employees having experienced bullying within the workplace (WBI, 2021).

Organizational Impact of Bullying

Organizations are impacted by bullying as well. Employees will leave an organization that does not have a healthy work environment (WBI, 2021). Hence, turnover intentions are likely to be higher and employee absences from the workplace increase. The reputation of the organization will be impacted over time and lawsuits may occur. As a result of poor branding and reputation, the organization will be unable to attract nor sustain talented workers. Because employees experience a disruption in their work as a result of the bullying and also a lack of confidence, productivity is impacted. Ultimately, the quality of customer service declines as costs to manage the organization and product(s) increase.

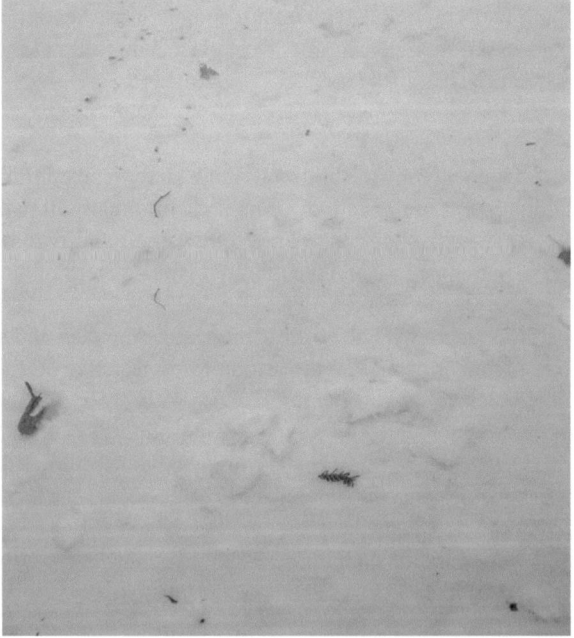

Cold

Cold Communications

Directions
For many people, responding to a rude or demeaning comment can be uncomfortable. However, at times, unaddressed untrue or negative behaviors can affect the health of the person being bullied. Additionally, addressing the unprofessional behaviors of a coworker(s) can help in the unit-based and organizational initiatives to create healthy work environments for all people. Read each statement and decide if you will respond, not respond, or be undecided. Answers will vary and depend upon an individual's personality and personal life experiences. Hence, below the questions are possible considerations only when responding.

Statement (bully) 1. "Sometimes I wonder if you really have a brain."
Response (affected person) 1. "I am certain that I do. I met the qualifications to work here just like you."
Select your response:
  (a) Respond.
  (b) Not respond.
  (c) Undecided.
Answer: Respond. It is important to set clear boundaries as to who you are and do not allow the bully to define you or your abilities.

Statement (bully) 2. "Let me explain how this works to ensure you understand."
Response (affected person) 2. No response.
Select your response:
  (a) Respond.
  (b) Not respond.
  (c) Undecided.
Answer: Not respond. This statement does not warrant a response. Some comments by people attempting to be rude or belittling to you are just not worth your energy. Maintain direct eye contact for a few moments with a neutral expression and drop your gaze. The latter demonstrates that their statement was meaningless to you and that you have already moved on to the next best thing.

Statement (bully) 3. (Insert name) "It looks like _____ is the last pick for project teams again. Anyone interested in _____ joining your team? What? Afraid of having to do "extra" work?"
Response (affected person) 2. "I enjoy working in teams and will do my best to help my team succeed. My work ethic is to arrive early and stay late."
Select your response:
  (a) Respond.
  (b) Not respond.
  (c) Undecided.
Answer: Respond. Reframe the negative statement with a positive one.

Statement (bully) 4. "That hairstyle you are wearing is very unprofessional. Braids and afros do not belong in the workplace."

Response (affected person) 4. "Have you ever heard of the Crown Act. You may want to read about this Act before you decide to make any more comments about my hair. Not appropriate."

Select your response:
(a) Respond.
(b) Not respond.
(c) Undecided.

Answer: Respond. It is important to recognize your own uniqueness and beauty as being valuable. No one has the right to disrespect who you are and how you choose to present yourself.

Statement (bully) 5. "Do you really think they will believe you… that all this was your idea. Look at me and then look at you?"

Response (affected person) 5. No response.

Select your response:
(a) Respond.
(b) Not respond.
(c) Undecided.

Answer: Not respond. No response is necessary to the bully; instead follow up with substantiating the origins of your work. It is your work and no one has the right to take credit for it but you.

Activity: Poof!

Meditation for Contemplation.

Poof!

Quietly lying in bed again but wide awake, I meditate on the failures of my own interventions to stop the bullying.

Tossing and turning. Repetition of words said and words I wish I could unsay; the determination of assigned fault seems relentless.

Scarred more than I care to admit I ruminate.

I ruminate over words said to me and words said about me.

The strength now emerging is not one of fantasy but of reality. This is my reality.

Mood uplifted and strength renewed, I awake to peace. What happened?

Poof!

I awoke from my toil. Tired of the endless and relentless nonsense of the bullies, I arose.

Stronger and unscathed.

Poof!

Meditation and Contemplation After reading the poetic meditation entitled "Poof!," consider how it made you feel. Answer the questions below.

1. What is the meaning of the title "Poof!"?
2. Why does the person in the poem have sleepless nights?
3. What made the person in the poem meditate on their own failures?
4. What causes a person to ruminate?
5. What causes a person to have their strength renewed?

References

Green, C. (2019). *Incivility among nursing professionals in clinical and academic environments: Emerging research and opportunities*. IGI Global. https://doi.org/10.4018/978-1-5225-7341-8. ISBN 13: 9781522573418.

Green, C. (2020). The hollow: A theory on workplace bullying in nursing practice. *Nursing Forum, 56*(1). https://doi.org/10.1111/nuf.12539

Heinrich, K. (2007). Joy stealing: 10 mean games faculty play and how to stop the gaming. *Nurse Educator, 32*(1), 34–38. https://journals.lww.com/nurseeducatoronline/Abstract/2007/01000/Joy_Stealing__10_Mean_Games_Faculty_Play_and_How.10.aspx

Park, M., & Choi, J. S. (2019). Effects of workplace cyberbullying on nurses' symptom experience and turnover intention. *Journal of Nursing Management, 27*(6), 1108–1115. https://doi.org/10.1111/jonm.12779

Praslova, L. N., Carucci, R., & Stokes, C. (2022). How bullying manifests at work–and how to stop it. *Harvard Business Review*. https://hbr.org/2022/11/how-bullying-manifests-at-work-and-how-to-stop-it

The Guardian. (2014). Rude boys: Shanty Town to Savile Row. https://www.theguardian.com/artanddesign/2014/may/24/rude-boys-jamaican-subculture-photography-exhibition

Underground Music, Art, & Subculculture (2021, March 1). *The story of subculture: The rude boy (and rude girl)*. https://underground-england.com/the-story-of-subculture-the-rude-boy-rude-girl/

Valclavikova, K., & Kozakova, R. (2022). Mobbing and its effects on the health of a selected sample of nurses in The Czech Republic. *Nursing in the 21st Century, 21*(1), 29–33. https://doi.org/10.2478/pielxxiw-2022-0008

Workplace Bullying Institute. (2021). *2021 WBI workplace bullying survey*. https://workplacebullying.org/2021-wbi-survey/

Structured Workplace Chaos   3

Learning Objectives

1. Explain how structured workplace chaos can negatively impact workplace cultures if unaddressed by organizations.
2. Describe how employees can become advocates for change in dysfunctional workplaces.
3. Decipher ways in which nurses affected by structured workplace chaos can maintain professional and emotional integrity.

Introduction

Dysfunction is defined two ways by the Merriam-Webster Online Dictionary: as an actual impairment in abnormal functioning and a person or persons unhealthy interaction(s) within a group or interpersonal behavior(s) (Merriam-Webster Online Dictionary, 2024). When bullying is ignored within the workplace environment, a healthy environment of collegiality and mutual respect cannot be maintained. Under the hidden guise of smiles at a team meeting lie hidden inappropriate temperaments, fabrication of information, and low-level sarcasm. The response of the closed-off and dysfunctional team dynamic is silence. An occasional question that may challenge the abnormal is met with dismissal by the bully or bullies within the group.

Workplace dysfunction is able to permeate workplaces when leadership is afraid or consciously decides not to address their bullying problem. Unfortunately, organizations will be impacted by the bullying via turnover intentions, reduced productivity, and lawsuits. Employees can be proactive in the promotion of change, but many in the protection of their own health and wellness make the healthy decision to leave their dysfunctional workplaces.

This dysfunction within workplace teams does not happen overnight but has been sustained for years to decades because anyone who challenges the dysfunction is met with actual roadblocks occurring within multiple levels within the organization. Interestingly enough, some workplaces choose to intentionally maintain dysfunction because it does not have to make progressive changes for its customers or workers. Of concern is that this level of dysfunction in healthcare environments can lead to patients dying and no one taking accountability as families mourn and healthcare workers with a conscious who care about positive and progressive change, leave their jobs. Hence, the cycle continues.

Dysfunctional units, divisions, schools, and departments can exist in any workplace environment. Dysfunction is the lived experience of confusion, disruption, corruption, lies, thievery, and selective self-righteousness that seeks to destroy one, a few, or many for the sole purpose of gaining power. Hence, when dysfunction arises in workplaces, the only solution to end the dysfunction is to expose it and those that perpetrate its delusion. Dysfunction will only persist to exist when ignored and accepted as being a reality, and not fallacy.

Hypothetical Case Study: "That Is Not True!"

Another dysfunctional staff meeting. An agenda focused on upholding fallacy. Sally was the type of person who had a difficult time acknowledging her weaknesses and failures. Errors would never be acknowledged but blamed on other colleagues. Trudy listened to Sally's words and watched her in disbelief. Sally's mouth curved and twisted and she stated angrily, "That is not true!" Then, as if well-rehearsed within a theatre class, Sally began to cry in absence of tears.

Trudy thought to herself, "I cannot be the only one that sees that Sally's behavior is unprofessional and that she has once again got away with blaming her poor work performance on others." Trudy searched the room, curious if her colleagues had just heard and saw what Sally had just verbalized. Her colleagues' eyes, as they met hers, trailed off looking out windows, staring down at the ground, or pretending to read an empty page of notes. One colleague shook their head in total disbelief and then shrugged her shoulders in silence.

When the meeting ended, no one said anything to Trudy; it was as if nothing had occurred. One staff member went to console Sally. It was all so surreal. Only three people appeared in Trudy's office after the staff meeting to acknowledge the truth of what had occurred. Thirty healthcare professionals had been present at the meeting.

Groupthink

Groupthink occurs when people collaborate to reach a consensus on a specific subject matter(s). When groupthink occurs within workplace settings, individual creativity and ideas are not recognized. Persons find it easier or less stressful to agree with a group of people, rather than debate specific ideology brought forth by individuals that are a part of the group itself (Cha et al., 2020). Groupthink played a part in Trudy's colleagues not responding to the dysfunction that they had chosen to not address. In this case, the "group" decided that by not addressing the issue, they avoided becoming a part of the problem.

Territorialism

Green and Dimino Luong (2023), in discussing the concept of territorialism, noted that both formal and informal leaders within organizations that have exhibited bullying behaviors often have historically done so and use their knowledge of the organization to positively and negatively impact others. The fear of loss of perceived power and loss of control drives the employees who embody territorialism to bully others. In order to disrupt the bully who uses territorialism to stand their ground in their familiar department or unit, changing their environment and co-workers can be the start of the end of their reign.

Sabotage

Sabotage is a well-planned conspiracy theory practiced and executed for the sole purpose of physically attacking or emotionally harming another. Nurses can observe workplace dysfunction when communicating with co-workers who bully, patients, other healthcare workers, and patient's families. However, the direct observation of bullying does not mean that the observance will translate to action to prevent the bullying from occurring. The latter requires nurses to address their own fears of retaliation by the bully or bullies and to confidently go against the normal comfort zone of groupthink.

Interestingly, a room filled with nurses who have at one point in their careers cared and advocated for their fellow human beings (patients/clients), and yet in the presence of a bullying mob of colleagues, choose to be powerless in helping one another. The decision to be motionless and silent when witnessing bullying perpetuates dysfunction. The latter empowers bullies and worsens the toxicity in the workplace.

An example of sabotage in practice:

The Depleted Nurse

Baffled by their own inability to speak up at times when confronted with workplace bullying, nurses, in the course of their education to become nurses, become embattled and fatigued. Nurses must learn to become "highly skilled health care workers" in a matter of a few years. Be it a 1-, 2-, 3- or 4-year program of academic study and clinical practice exposure, the ever-growing content of healthcare seems endless, and prelicensure nurses are overwhelmed. Nurses therefore enter the nursing profession emotionally depleted. Depleted of energy and at times fearful of the next challenge, it can seem easier for nurses to ignore dysfunction within their work environments than to speak up and help make positive changes.

Can't Do It

When working in a workplace that does not permit individual thriving and professional growth, change can feel unachievable. Employees become frustrated because of perceived challenges related to the resistance of change within workplaces they are employed. The status quo is quickly adopted within these work environments, and purposeful dysfunction develops. New ideology is dismissed, in favor of maintaining the status quo. In absence of productive and innovative change within work cultures, the emergence of toxic workplace environments can begin.

When highly motivated persons enter the workplace environment that has adapted to the status quo, they may attempt to introduce innovation and promote change. It is often these highly motivated individuals that are targeted by bullies who are fearful of change and intimidated by the persons that they perceive have become a disruption. Toxicity ensues as the employees who bully attempt to exert their perceived power in the workplace with the goal of discrediting another person.

For the person experiencing The Hollow, they tend to represent the highly motivated employee that is desirous of change and innovation. The latter is counterintuitive to the toxic work environment where there is often a power imbalance. As a result, the bully or bullies will utilize coercion skills like that of groupthink to dismantle any perceived power the employee desiring change has.

Structural Chaos in the Workplace

Structural chaos in the workplace is the planned constructed attempt to discredit and or minimize another's accomplishments. Structured chaos is created by the bully via lying, gossiping, and devaluing of another's creative works and or intellectual property. In addressing structural chaos, it is imperative that employees and leadership listen to affected persons to develop a clear timeline of when the structured chaos plan began and the attempt to discredit the affected person emerged. By identifying the timeline, key players of the bullying can be identified.

Structural Empowerment

Employees in the workplace can be empowered to voice their concerns or desire for proactive environmental and structural change through structured empowerment. **Structural empowerment** is a theory that explores both informal and formal allegiances between subordinates and superiors and networks of peer groups as means to influence positive changes in work culture and the organization. Employees that have formal power within an organization have roles that are aligned with organizational vision and mission statements that are flexible. Informal power roles are held by employees that maintain interpersonal relationships with employees at all levels within the organization, while themselves not holding a formal leadership position of formal power. Kanter (1977) noted that employees that are committed to the success of the organization seek for opportunities to grow professionally and have job satisfaction and will thrive in workplaces that support structural empowerment (Laschinger et al., 2001).

Incivility

Uncivil conduct in the academic and workplace environments occurs when employees experience the negative behaviors of a bully or group of bullies. The bully or group of bullies may be a co-worker, supervisor, administrator, or an employee at any level within the hierarchy of the organization. The uncivil conduct manifests itself as incivility. **Incivility** is demonstrated by discourteousness, rude behaviors directed at others for the primary purpose of humiliation and disruption of a person or persons' lives. According to Einarsen et al. (2009) person-related incivility, physical intimidation, and work-related incivility are the three most common types of incivility. The complexity of incivility in its manifestation of lying, gossiping, belittlement, gaslighting, intimidation, and many other negative manipulative behaviors is that unaddressed, an unhealthy environment is left to proliferate. Hence, bullying worsens, and affected and unaffected bystanders who witness the incivility feel unsupported and vulnerable.

Unaffected bystander vulnerability in witnessed incivility is the result of persons who witness co-worker(s) (or fellow student(s)) being bullied and consciously decide not to intervene for fear of becoming a victim of the bully or bullies themselves. The unaffected bystander's fear leads them to deny the existence of the occurrence(s) of incivility though witnessed by them. As a result, unaffected bystanders reject or avoid the person or persons being bullied. The unaffected bystander may also deny the existence of bullying behaviors actually occurring to managers, administrators, and Human Resource Department representatives. The sole purpose of the behavior of the unaffected bystander is self-protection. The unaffected bystander is afraid of becoming a victim themselves, of the bully or bullies.

Summary

There are several factors impacting employees and their co-worker relationships within the workplace. Healthy workplaces welcome new ideas and the employees who share them. The maintaining of the status quo is not as important as innovation and change, because the organizational goal is productivity. Toxic workplaces can impair productivity because groupthink or individual control is prioritized over individual thought and willpower. In the support of healthy workplaces and employees, structured workplace chaos must be disarmed and ended. Failure to do so will result in employee burnout and increased turnover intentions.

Examples of Structured Workplace Chaos

Directions Read each of the two structured workplace chaos case studies and discuss what in the case studies points to negative behaviors that have been permitted to flourish within the work environment.

Case Study 1
Mitchell never says hello when he enters the office. His office colleagues have to await to determine how his mood is and if it's "safe" to share a greeting. It is clearly understood by everyone that it is wise to use caution before initiating a conversation. Awaiting for Mitchell to talk is always the "best" move.

Case Study 2
Margaret never meets deadlines, so none of the teams at work want to work with her. Margaret is known to "never carry her load." Kevin, Margaret's boss, is aware of Margaret's poor work performance but does nothing to address her less than desirable work habits. Lately, Margaret's co-workers have been discussing their lack of motivation to "work well and with purpose" given that low performance is acceptable in their workplace.

Activity: Identification of Bully Roles and Hidden Agendas in the Workplace Environment

Workplace Scenarios

Directions Read each scenario and determine what is the strategic role of the bully and the bully's hidden agenda within the workplace. Determine the role of witnesses to the acts of bullying when applicable to the scenario, as well. Circle the answer. Discuss with peers why you selected your answer before discussing the correct answer.

Scenario 1 Adam was quiet as he sat in the staff lounge eating his lunch overhearing Michael and Benjamin barrage Franklin. Franklin had recently received an award for his excellence in the delivery of patient care and recognition of subtle signs and symptoms of patients' condition deterioration and his active participation in rapid responses that led to the saving of the lives of at least six patients in the past 8 months. Franklin, a medical-surgical nurse, had aspirations to become a nurse anesthetist, and his next career move within the coming year was to transfer to a critical care unit.

The barrage that Adam witnessed his colleague Franklin receive was nearly unbearable to watch. Michael and Benjamin cursed at him, called him a "suck up," a "failure as a nurse," "disliked by most co-workers," and proceeded to pour their cups of coffee over his sandwich and salad that he was having for lunch. Adam stood up from a chair he was sitting in finishing up his own lunch, made minimal eye contact with Franklin, and, in silence, walked away. On the clinical unit, when Franklin returned to resume the care of his patients, he was visibly shaken and had a difficult time concentrating. While Adam felt bad about what he had witnessed happen to Franklin, he in no way wanted to be involved. So, Adam decided not to discuss the incident with Franklin or anyone else.

Scenario 1 Discussion: Let's talk about this…

1. The strategic role of the bullies and their hidden agenda in Scenario 1 was to demean the achievements of another person through sharing falsehoods and discredit the person's accomplishments.
2. Adam's response was no response. Adam intentionally made the decision to not get involved and, instead, watched Franklin be bullied. Adam acted in fear. His fear was of becoming a victim himself of bullying, if he involved himself in the situation.
3. Michael and Benjamin likely have been bullying others for quite some time. Their responses exhibit confidence and clarity in their expression of dislike for their target—Franklin.
4. Franklin feels exposed as he notices Adam is present in the staff lounge. Franklin's response is the internalization of words and actions that are emotionally hurtful and targeted toward him by Michael and Benjamin. The exposure of being bullied can be crippling as the affected person can feel helpless and hopeless in their situation. Bodily, they are fatigued and lack energy in other areas of their lives because being bullied is emotionally draining.

Scenario 1 Questions:

1. Should Adam have attempted to engage Franklin in a conversation to remove him from the bullying situation?
2. Did Adam make the right decision to not talk to Michael or Benjamin about their negative interaction with Franklin?
3. Is it difficult to observe another person be treated unfairly by someone else?
4. If you were Adam, what would be your next steps after returning to the clinical unit to resume your work?

Scenario 2 Jessica had changed jobs to spend more time with her family and at home resting. The last 5 months had been difficult because she had to take a leave of absence to take care of her husband who was dying of lung cancer. Jessica felt depressed and isolated. She had been married to her husband for 25 years and was now left to raise their 10-year-old son alone.

Jessica was well-known in her company as a "fixer." Fixers are synonymous with repairing dysfunctional workplace environments once recognized by administration as being problematic. Examples of dysfunctional workplace environments that a "fixer" would be requested to implement change within include those work environments having decreased productivity, high turnover intentions, and poor patient health outcomes. Jessica's reputation as a "fixer" had led to her quickly rising to the level of Executive Director within 3 years of working within the company after entering the health system in the role of clinical nurse specialist.

Jessica was kind and considerate to her co-workers and a strong advocate for patients entering the health system to receive care. When Jessica returned to work, she took the position of a part-time 24-h staff nurse on a stroke rehabilitation unit. Jessica took the part-time nursing position to ensure that she was available to be home with her son in the evening to support him with homework and maintain a regular schedule of family time together. Jessica enjoyed working as a bedside nurse leader and was excited to be involved in the day-to-day care of patients and educating patients and their families about various medications, conditions, and disease processes.

Melinda was a night shift nurse who recently changed her alternating work weekends and weekly schedule to accommodate her return to graduate school. Melinda instantly recognized Jessica as being the Executive Director who had thwarted her plans to return to graduate school 2 years ago. Melinda approached Jessica angrily and said, "Oh, it's you. Whose life are you trying to mess up now?" Jessica, who encountered many nurses in her role as a nurse leader, did not recognize Melinda at all. Jessica, looking at Melinda with a smirk on her face, stated, "Am I supposed to know you?"

Melinda shared with peers her interaction with Jessica and her previous role within the organization. Melinda and her co-workers, some who also had negative experiences with Jessica in her nurse leader role, began to sabotage her work, spread rumors, and would not assist her when she required help in the provision of care to her patients. Jessica, realizing that she had become a target of bullying in the workplace, met with her manager to complain and report Melinda as the primary perpetrator.

Scenario 2 Discussion: Let's talk about this…

1. Jessica's transition to a direct care position provided additional family time with her 10-year-old son. The career transition occurred around Jessica becoming a widow. Life transitions can be both positive and negative. Because this was the loss of a spouse that then led to a career change and self-demotion, it is likely that Jessica may be experiencing multiple losses.
2. Sometimes after significant losses, the affected person(s) may desire to be "unseen." To be "unseen" is to be unrecognizable and to "fly below the radar." Jessica's decision to return to bedside nursing provided a way to leave behind the demands of an Executive Director position and focus on physical and emotional healing.

3. Melinda's recognition of Jessica as the person who had disrupted her academic studies while she was actively pursuing a graduate degree likely brought about feelings of frustration, anger, and betrayal.
 4. Melinda, seeing that her former boss was now a co-worker, decidedly took action to bully Jessica to seek revenge.

Scenario 2 Questions

 1. Why did Jessica make the decision to demote herself at work?
 2. What was Melinda's history with Jessica?
 3. Did Jessica's response to Melinda warrant the bullying?
 4. Could the entire situation have been avoided?
 5. What can the manager of the unit do to remedy this situation?
 6. Can bullying be passed on as a behavior that is reciprocal when more than one party is injured?
 7. In the case of Jessica and Melinda, are both persons equally at fault of unprofessional conduct within the workplace?
 8. Should Melinda be disciplined?
 9. Should Jessica be held accountable for her past actions, all be it in a different role, within the organization?
 10. Should organizational standards of conduct be reinforced by the unit manager?

Scenario 3 Michael was both a scoundrel and a gentleman. He knew when to schmooze and when to lay low. None of the team trusted him. Michael was known to lie and align with anyone who could possibly bring him accolades with minimal effort on his part. Hence, Michael had a keen eye for talent that made him shine brightly in the eyes of administration.

When Florence joined Michael's team of clinical outcome leaders, she had already been a well-established administrator for 25 years and a statistician for 15 years. Florence simply wanted to retire in 4 years without the burden of "work being taken home." Michael met with Florence and gave her one project to initiate unto completion. The project examined the surgical outcomes of cardiac transplant patients regarding complications of surgical site infections within 30 days of the procedure.

Florence was excited to begin the project. The project lasted 10 weeks, and an additional 4 weeks were taken to tabulate and examine the statistical evidence. Florence presented the project results to Michael and other key stakeholders within the organization. Michael then asked Florence to begin writing the manuscript describing the project's purpose, process, and outcome for submission to journals. When the manuscript was completed, Florence submitted the manuscript to Michael for review.

After having the manuscript for 6 weeks, Florence asked to return it to her so she can begin submitting the manuscript. Michael shared that he had submitted the manuscript to a journal 5-weeks ago and would be likely hearing from the journal in another 5 weeks, on the status of the manuscript. Florence was disappointed and hurt. However, Florence also felt that as a team member, Michael's submission of the project ultimately was for the benefit of the organization and all those who participated in the project: patients, physicians, patient care associates (e.g., nurse assistants), nursing staff, and surgical technicians.

Fast forward 4 weeks later, the manuscript was accepted by a cardiology journal. When published 3 months later, the publication's sole author was Michael. Florence, the Principal Investigator and her many Co-investigators of physicians, nurses, patient care associates (e.g., nurse assistants), and surgical technicians were not given credit for their work. Their names were excluded from the manuscript. Florence had the difficult task of explaining to her research team, how their hard work was not given credit as promised.

Scenario 3 Discussion: Let's talk about this…

1. Michael's history of dishonesty was seemingly ignored by Florence. Perhaps she desired to give him a chance to prove himself different despite of what was rumored and discussed about him by his colleagues within the organization.
2. Florence and her fellow research team members' talents were exploited.
3. Taking credit for another's work benefits no one.

Scenario 3 Questions

1. Why was Florence assigned the research project by Michael?
2. Should Michael apologize to Florence and the research team?
3. Did Michael plagiarize by not giving credit to other's work? If yes, could disciplinary action be taken against him?
4. What was the sole purpose of Michael's actions?

Activities Acknowledging Workplace Ingenuity

Recognizing Healthy and Not So Healthy Workplace Communication Responses

Directions Read the following ten examples of workplace communications, and determine which are healthy communications and unhealthy communications.

1. "I thought what you said was not very clear. You just seemed very uncomfortable."
2. "Your oral skills need some work. You do a lot of repeating of the same information when you are nervous."
3. "The flow of your paper requires some revising. Have you considered hiring an Editor?"
4. "The ideas you come up with are really off the mark. I think we should meet to get you back on the right track."

5. "Let's have a vote. Who thought Sarah's speech was good?"
6. "What you just said makes no sense?"
7. "We will be taking over the project anyway."
8. "An excellent idea. Let's get together to develop it further as a team."
9. "Wow, it is evident that you have been working really hard on this project Bob."
10. "You have been eating up a lot of company time Judy. Why is this job seemingly so hard for you?"

Answers

Recognizing Healthy and Not So Healthy Workplace Communication Responses

Directions Read the following ten examples of workplace communications, and determine which are healthy communications and unhealthy communications.

1. "I thought what you said was not very clear. You just seemed very uncomfortable."
    healthy communications or **unhealthy communications**
2. "Your oral skills need some work. You do a lot of repeating of the same information when you are nervous."
    healthy communications or **unhealthy communications**
3. "The flow of your paper requires some revising. Have you considered hiring an Editor?"
    healthy communications or **unhealthy communications**
4. "The ideas you come up with are really off the mark. I think we should meet to get you back on the right track."
    healthy communications or **unhealthy communications**
5. "Let's have a vote. Who thought Sarah's speech was good?"
    healthy communications or **unhealthy communications**
6. "What you just said makes no sense?"
    healthy communications or **unhealthy communications**
7. "We will be taking over the project anyway."
    healthy communications or **unhealthy communications**
8. "An excellent idea. Let's get together to develop it further as a team."
    healthy communications or unhealthy communications
9. "Wow, it is evident that you have been working really hard on this project Bob."
    healthy communications or unhealthy communications
10. "You have been eating up a lot of company time Judy. Why is this job seemingly so hard for you?"
    healthy communications or **unhealthy communications.**

Activity

Identification of Mindsets

Directions Read each of the five sets of two mindsets presented, and select one of the two mindsets presented. Answer the questions below:

1. Who are you? Mindset 1 or Mindset 2?
2. Why is the truth important?
3. What does it mean to be transparent?
4. Why is it easy to lie instead of honoring the good in others?

Mindset 1
Mindset 1: "I know you believe in transparency but it can paint the liar as a liar. I prefer to pretend that I am coherent to the truth and more absorbent of that which is not always accurate. That's my preference in communication. I know it is ineffective, but it is purposeful because I can use distraction to avoid doing my job."
Mindset 2: The truth is important because it can bring a peaceful end to altercations and lead to respectful speech and honorable listening skills.

Mindset 2
Mindset 1: "This is hard. How can I work in an environment that is so volatile? I never know when I am going to be verbally attacked."
Mindset 2: "There are volatile people in many of life's situations that can occur daily. In traffic or within lines at the grocery store. The behaviors of volatile people are not mine. I do not have to own other's bad behaviors."

Mindset 3
Mindset 1: "Loneliness in the workplace is real when people deem you to be different."
Mindset 2: "Diversity in the workplace brings a richness that is important to us and to those persons we interact with."

Mindset 4
Mindset 1: "The habitual pattern of negative self-talk can destroy the morale of all persons in its path."
Mindset 2: "What comes out of my mouth has no effect on me or those around me."

Mindset 5
Mindset 1: "Mental emptiness is the process of purging the mind from thoughts that are not productive."
Mindset 2: "Selflessness is the purging of selfishness and making the conscious decision to actually care for others."

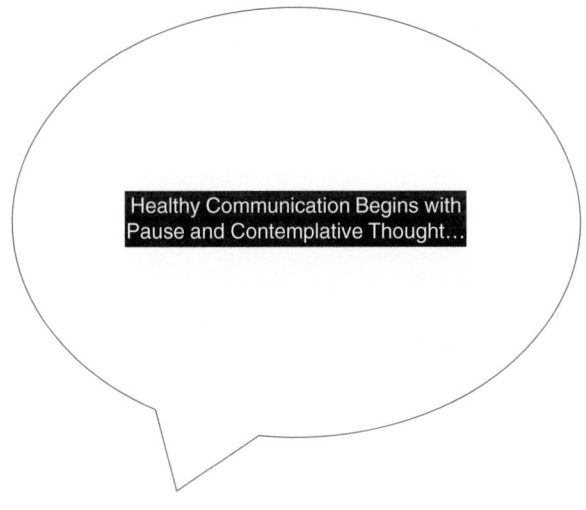

References

Cha, N., Hwang, J., & Kim, E. (2020). The optimal knowledge creation strategy of organizations in groupthink situations. *Computational & Mathematical Organization Theory, 26*(2), 207–235. https://doi-org.acu.idm.oclc.org/10.1007/s10588-020-09313-w

Einarsen, S., Hoel, H., & Notelaers, G. (2009). Measuring exposure to bullying and harassment at work: Validity, factor structure and psychometric properties of the negative acts questionnaire—Revised. *Work & Stress: An International Journal of Work, Health & Organisations, 23*(1), 24–44. https://doi.org/10.1080/02678370902815673

Green, C., & Dimino Luong, A. (2023). Bullied: Exploring the concepts of territorialism and groupthink involvement in workplace bullying. *Nursing Open, 10*(10), 6777–6781. https://doi.org/10.1002/nop2.1938

Kanter, R. (1977). *Men and women of the corporation*. Basic Books.

Laschinger, H. K. S., Finegan, J. M., Shamian, J., & Wilk, P. (2001). Impact of structural and psychological empowerment on job strain in nursing work settings: Expanding Kanter's model. *Journal of Nursing Administration, 31*(5), 260–272. https://doi.org/10.1097/00005110-200105000-00006

Merriam Webster Online Dictionary. (2024). *Dysfunction*. https://www.merriam-webster.com/dictionary/dysfunction

Patients Matter

4

Learning Objectives

1. Describe the origin of the word patient.
2. Explain how healthcare organizations facilitate the initiation of healthcare for patients entering their systems.
3. Discuss the role of the nurse as the protector of the patient.
4. Examine the importance of patient-centered healthcare.

Introduction

According to medical sociologist, the assuming of the role of patient involves the forfeiting of certain freedoms. Personal clothing is replaced with a hospital gown referred to as a "johnny" that allows for immediate access to the human body by healthcare workers and providers for physical examinations, assessments, placement of intravenous (IV) access for delivery of IV fluids and medications, and diagnostic tests (e.g., X-rays, ultrasounds, PET scans, etc.). Persons assume the role of "patient" after accepting that something is potentially not physically or emotionally well within themselves (Frank, 2013; Parsons, 1951; Schipke, 2021).

Patients

The word **patient** originates from the Latin *patiens* or *patior* meaning one who bears or suffers (Neuberger, 1999). Historically, the role of patient is one of passivity. Illness, mental and physical, happens to the patient and is uninvited. The unpredictability of the sick role experience is what has linked the patient role not with empowerment within the healthcare system but dependence and vulnerability. However, just because one adapts to their surroundings' use of language (e.g., medical terminology), dress, and conduct does not mean that they are disempowered. Adaptation for functionality does not always equate to lack of access or knowledge of one's illness state. It is also important to note that not all patients enter healthcare systems ill but for wellness checks to maintain health.

The vulnerability of patients occurs when there is no inquiry involved in their interfacing with the healthcare system. When information about illness and diseases one is diagnosed with is not provided by healthcare workers or healthcare providers, it is then that the patient role becomes one that is at risk for poor treatment and health outcomes. Hence, health disparities can occur within the patient role related to language barriers, race, socioeconomics, gender, ability to read and comprehend the medical information, sex, and other factors (Green, 2021).

Healthcare Organizations

Healthcare organizations are structurally designed systems that are built with the intent to provide healthcare services in designated locations with varied populations. Healthcare organizations can include a physician group practice associated with a hospital system, clinics, hospitals, a host of different types of healthcare disciplines (e.g., nurses, physical therapists, respiratory therapists, physicians, etc.), third-party payers, the insured, specialty boards, and medical specialty groups (Agency for Healthcare Research and Quality, 2023). Additional services provided by healthcare organizations are home care, subacute care (e.g., skilled nursing facilities), acute care, hospice, and palliative care.

Healthcare organizations have become larger in size and have been purchasing multiple hospitals and building several clinics and urgent care facilities to address outpatient service public demands. When healthcare organizations are associated with academic institutions, research and evidenced-based practice are emphasized as being integrated into projected health outcomes for patient populations treated within the organizations. In order for populations residing in communities surrounding healthcare organizations to have their healthcare needs adequately met, healthcare organizations must invest in the investigation of risk factors associated with mortality and morbidity.

Patient-Centered Healthcare

Patient-centered healthcare involves putting the patient and their physiological, psychological, and spiritual needs first. By embracing the patient first approach, all environmental and policy decisions related to patients are a priority. With the patient-centered care approach, theoretically, health systems exist solely to meet the needs of men, women, infants, and children who enter and exit the doors of their facilities. According to Santana et al. (2018), patient-centered care itself is conceptually a holistic approach that is inclusive, empowering, individualized, and respectful of all persons. Caregiver leaders within healthcare organizations place their own personal relationship with patients as a priority, especially when planning and delivering patient health care.

Healthcare workers enter the field of healthcare to contribute to the identification, diagnosis, and implementation of care for ill patients. Ill patients drive the dedicated healthcare worker to make a difference not only in their lives but in the lives of others. Hence, patient-centered care is not a formidable task but a natural occurrence for healthcare workers, such as nurses who have made the conscious decision to enter professions providing care to persons suffering from physical and mental illnesses.

The Assumption of Sick Role

Talcott Parsons, a sociologist practicing within the United States, developed the theory of social systems. The social systems theory (Parsons, 1951) explores the various roles held in society and the expectations placed on these roles and the persons who assume them in varied situations. The *sick role*, one of the roles identified by Parsons (Parsons, 1975), is assumed by persons once labeled with an illness or diagnosis.

The assumption of the sick role often begins by the person acknowledging that their health status has changed. Physical and or mental symptomatology overcomes the affected person's mind and body. The affected person will either present to a healthcare facility such as an urgent care center, a doctor's office, community-based clinic, or emergency department within an acute care hospital setting to seek help.

Stripped of one's own clothing, the sick person is welcomed into the health system with the changing into a disposable or cloth gown. The gown allows for ease of access for healthcare providers and healthcare workers to examine and assess the sick person using devices such as a stethoscope, the accessing of the veins (or arteries) to obtain blood specimens, ultrasounds, X-rays, or computed tomography (CT) scans. The process of diagnosis ensues as data is gathered via procedures, assessments, and evaluations. Ultimately, with critical analysis of gathered historical and past medical and surgical information, a diagnosis or diagnoses are made.

Lastly, with a known cause of illness or disease origination, the person in the sick role either accepts the proposed treatment or denies help. The engagement or disengagement with the healthcare system is the choice of the affected person. Their decision can have either lifesaving results, stabilization with cure, or the acceptance of a poor prognosis depending upon the diagnostic outcome projection made by healthcare providers, hence, the acceptance of death.

Nurses and Patients

Nurses exhibit caritas toward their patients by meeting their physical, emotional, and spiritual needs. The assessment, diagnosis, planning, interventions, and evaluations performed by nurses for their patients literally stabilize disease processes, contribute to the diagnostic process, and save lives. The therapeutic foundations of the nurse-patient relationship develop with the initial communication of greeting and nurses' introduction of themselves and their role in the provision of care to the patient. In academic nursing programs, nursing students are introduced to the concept of communication as a means to share and exchange information while transmitting and generating meaning. The latter occurs between two or more persons (Taylor et al., 2023).

Forms of Communication

Communication involves the sending and receiving of both verbal and nonverbal communication by nurses and the patients in their care. Within verbal communication, language must be interpreted if the two persons do not share the same cultural and or geographic background. For nonverbal communication, the concepts of time and space will vary among persons of different cultures. Additionally, the way one moves their body, makes eye contact, and maintains boundaries are all impacted by their personal life experiences, culture, and any deficits in kinesthetic, auditory, or visual transmission (Andrews et al., 2020).

In the process of applying the *nursing process* to clinical practice, nurses are taught during their undergraduate education to formulate patient care plans. One of the tools used in several academic settings is the nursing diagnosis applying the North American Nursing Diagnosis Association-International (NANDA-I). The NANDA-I provides a formal definition and defining characteristics of identified patient's risk factors (Ackley et al., 2022), related factors, potential outcomes, and evidenced-based and clinically appropriate nursing interventions with rationales that support the reason for and necessity of implementation of interventions in the provision of quality and safe nursing care.

Current communication nursing diagnoses include communication and communication problems that are defined based upon specific patient needs, deficits, and disease factors or illnesses contributing to lack of communication or an inability to communicate suggestive of an impairment. The latter is determined by the clinical and critical thinking of the nursing professional, in the context of exercising clinical judgment. The following are two areas of communication to be addressed:

1. Impaired verbal communication.
2. Readiness for enhanced communication.

Readiness for enhanced communication involves the verbal exchange of information with others. The exchange of information includes comprehension of another's thoughts, feelings, and objectives in the message they are delivering to another person. Communication, in absence of a language barrier or speech impediment, is understood by both parties. Impaired verbal communication is the absence, delay, or decrease in an individual's ability to use a system of symbols, transmit, receive, or process information. Characteristically, examples of impairment in verbal communication can include slurred speech associated with a brain injury, stroke, facial paralysis, selective inattention, absence of eye contact, hearing impairment, or muteness (Ackley et al., 2022; Newton & Shah, 2013).

Interpersonal Theory

Peplau (1952) examined the nurse-patient relationship with regard to the importance of the effectiveness of that which is being communicated and the clarity of the communication.

The Value of Effective Communication

Effective communication is invaluable because it constitutes the mutual listening, comprehension, and understanding of another person. Nurses, in their communication with patients, must demonstrate professionalism but most importantly, empathy and respect while nonjudgmentally gathering healthcare history and performing an assessment on their patients. Communication is necessary in the formation of therapeutic nurse-patient alliances that lead to diagnostic collaborations with healthcare providers and other disciplines in ensuring that patients are accurately diagnosed.

The Angry Patient

Patients enter healthcare environments under duress. Unexpected illnesses that require the intervention of healthcare workers place ill persons in a position of vulnerability and powerlessness as they wait in waiting rooms to be evaluated and undergo diagnostic tests. Patients are also asked to tell their "health decline" stories over and over again the moment they enter healthcare environments. While it is imperative that patients' past health histories be known in order for disease processes and illnesses to be identified, the repetition of "health decline" stories can heighten anxiety, increase fear, and frustrate patients. As a result of the latter, patients can become angry in their communications with nurses and other healthcare workers and professionals.

Workplace violence involving nurses is often perpetuated against them by patients, their families, or significant others. According to Lim et al. (2022), violence in the workplace can include threats and acts of violence such as harassment, verbal abuse, physical assault, homicide, or bullying. Physical violence incurred in the workplace can include slapping, kicking, gun violence, biting, stabbing, and pushing. Harassment is used as a way to verbally insult, bully, irritate, humiliate, intimidate, and degrade another person, while psychological violence involves the targeted use of power and threat of physical harm to impair the social, spiritual, physical, moral, and mental development of another person or persons. Approximately 73% of nonfatal illnesses and injuries in the workplace occurred due to workplace violence (United States Bureau of Labor Statistics, 2018). Over the course of their careers, 8–38% of healthcare workers are likely to experience physical violence (World Health Organization, 2022).

Summary

Because of the strong likelihood that working as a nurse interfacing with persons under duress, workplace violence can be encountered, the use of therapeutic nurse-patient communication is imperative. Maintaining space and boundaries, listening intently, avoiding prejudgments, and being respectful to all persons are necessary to the prevention of violence. Nurses must also be aware of protecting themselves in workplace situations that place them at risk for harm such as patients intoxicated with alcohol or under the influence of substances or involved in domestic violence or criminal acts in the community.

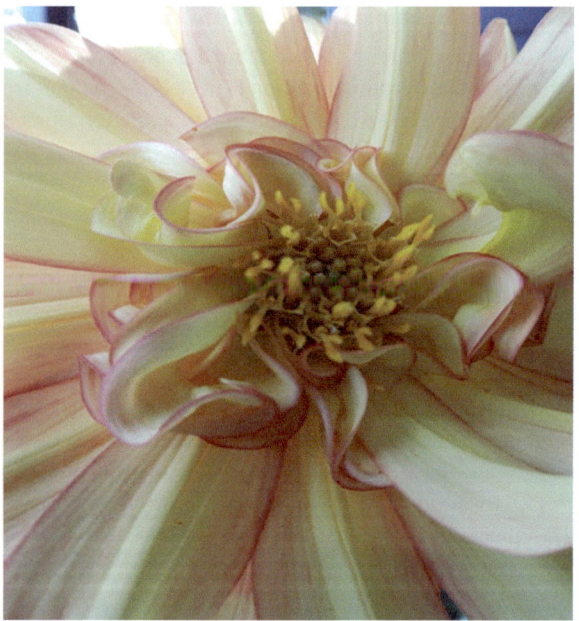

Delicate Beauty

References

Ackley, B. J., Ladwig, G. B., Flynn Makic, M. B., Martinez-Kratz, M., & Zanotti, M. (2022). *Nursing diagnosis handbook: An evidenced-based guide to planning care* (12th ed.). Elsevier.
Agency for Healthcare Research and Quality. (2023). *Defining health systems*. https://www.ahrq.gov/chsp/defining-health-systems/index.html

References

Andrews, M., Boyle, J. S., & Collins, J. (2020). *Transcultural concepts in nursing care* (8th ed.). Wolters Kluwer.

Frank, A. W. (2013). From sick role to practices of health and illness. *Medical Education, 47*(1), 18–25. https://doi.org/10.1111/j.1365-2923.2012.04298.x

Green, C. (2021). *Examining and solving health disparities in the United States: Emerging research and opportunities*. https://doi.org/10.4018/978-1-7998-3874-6. ISBN13: 9781799838746.

Lim, M. C., Jeffree, M. S., Saupin, S. S., Giloi, N., & Lukman, K. A. (2022). Workplace violence in healthcare settings: The risk factors, implications and collaborative preventive measures. *Annals of Medicine and Surgery, 78*. https://journals.lww.com/annals-of-medicine-and-surgery/fulltext/2022/06000/workplace_violence_in_healthcare_settings__the.29.aspx

Neuberger, J. (1999). Let's do away with "patients". *British Medical Journal, 318*(7200), 1756–1758. https://doi.org/10.1136/bmj.318.7200.1756

Newton, V. E., & Shah, S. R. (2013). Improving communication with patients with a hearing impairment. *Community Eye Health, 26*(81), 6–7. https://www.ncbi.nlm.nih.gov/pmc/articles/PMC3678307/

Parsons, T. (1951). *The social system*. Tavistock Publications.

Parsons, T. (1975). The sick role and the role of the physician reconsidered. The milbank memorial fund quarterly. *Health and Society, 53*, 257–278. https://doi.org/10.2307/3349493

Santana, M. J., Manalili, K., Jolley, R. J., Zelinsky, S., Quan, H., & Lu, M. (2018). How to practice person-centred care: A conceptual framework. *Health Expectations, 21*(2), 429–440. https://doi.org/10.1111/hex.12640

Schipke, T. (2021). The chronic sick role: Its time has come. *Omega: Journal of Death & Dying, 83*(3), 470–486. https://doi.org/10.1177/0030222819852848

Taylor, C., Lynn, P., & Barlett, J. L. (2023). *Fundamentals of nursing: The art and science of person-centered care* (10th ed.). Wolters Kluwer.

U.S. Bureau of Labour Statistics (USBLS). (2018). *Workplace violence in healthcare*. https://www.bls.gov/iif/oshwc/cfoi/workplace-violence-healthcare-2018.htm

World Health Organization (WHO). (2022). *Preventing violence against health workers*. https://www.who.int/activities/preventing-violence-against-health-workers

Unprovoked 5

Learning Objectives

1. Explain what it means to be involved in an unprovoked situation.
2. Discuss the effects of harming others, both intentionally and unintentionally.
3. Determine the potential benefits of healing oneself and discuss if healing oneself is possible.
4. Discuss how moving forward can bring closure.

Unprovoked

To be **unprovoked** in the workplace setting is to be involved in situations whereby there was seemingly no cause for what reportedly occurred to be validated or be reality-based. Hence, with regard to the bullying experience of The Hollow Theory, the bullied nurse is harassed without identifiable cause. And upon investigation the behaviors demonstrated by the bully or bullies is unjustifiable.

It is the unprovoked component of being bullied that confuses persons affected and targeted by the actual act of bullying. For persons experiencing The Hollow, it is the question of "Why this is happening to me?" that is ruminated upon both internally by the conscious and externally, verbally, as the person attempts to explain to others their encounters with the bully or bullies. The latter is why persons who are bullied, regardless of their level of intelligence, years of work experience, or accomplishments, tend to isolate and not share with others that they are being bullied, often waiting until the bullying has impacted their physical and emotional health and well-being.

Harming Others

Bullying harms others. While the bully or bullies have an intentional plan or purpose in the harming of their target(s), it is the unprovoked component of the bullying process that bewilders the affected person. Bullies are reliant upon their targets' response of bewilderment because it further arms them with the ability to harass inconspicuously. The **harming of others** is perpetuated when the bully or bullies seek to disarm others by verbally or physically targeting them within the work environment.

The Bewilderment of Gaslighting

The term *gaslighting* comes from a 1938 play entitled, "Angel Street" that was set in the year 1880 in London. The play was written by the playwright and British novelist, Patrick Hamilton. In the play, a married man uses subtle tricks to make his new wife gradually feel like she is going insane (Hamilton, 1966). The namesake of the tormenting trickery used by the spouse originates as he gradually dims the lights in their home that were "gas-fueled," hence, the origin of the term "gaslighting." The unsuspecting wife initially notices that the lights in the home have become dim, but as her seemingly innocent and well-intended husband denies that the gas-fueled lights have not dimmed, the wife begins to think she is losing her mind. Ironically, the story takes place on a street called Angel Street, which further alludes to the innocence and trust in angelic heavenly beings. Metaphorically, the person who gaslights is one who appears innocent and caring to others, while those that are being tricked by them are unaware of the gaslighter's trickery.

According to Feilding-Singh and Dmowska (2022), the goal of the gaslighter is to gradually cause the person they are targeting to develop self-doubt. The act of perpetuating self-doubt is implemented by the gaslighter through carefully crafting stories about the person that they are targeting that undermine their skillset and ability to perform their job. For example, a supervisor who is a gaslighter may say to an employee who has been excelling within their position at work, "I was talking to some of your peers and one of them said that your performance on the last project was not up to par like it has been in the past. Is something going on with you at home or work?" The gaslighter's inquiry about the target's personal and professional life is inappropriate and has no basis. However, the gaslighter uses this type of inquiry to create doubt and to cause the target to share private information that the gaslighter can strategically use to further undermine the target's performance at work.

The more frequent the incidences of gaslighting, the more the targeted person is psychologically impacted and begins to question their own abilities. However, targeted persons can experience a one-time incident with a gaslighter and be impacted (Johnson et al., 2021). The good news is that once the targeted person can recognize that they are being gaslighted, healing can begin.

Dominance

Dominance over the target is a win for the gaslighter. Gaslighters are believed to diagnostically exhibit the characteristics of a person with narcissistic personality disorder (Boring, 2020). The following is the diagnostic criteria for narcissistic personality disorder from the Diagnostic and Statistical Manual of Mental Disorders Fifth Edition (DSM-5):

Narcissistic Personality Disorder 301.81 (F60.81)

A pervasive pattern of grandiosity (in fantasy or behavior), need for admiration, and lack of empathy, beginning by early adulthood and present in a variety of contexts, as indicated by five (or more) of the following:

1. Has a grandiose sense of self-importance (e.g., exaggerates achievements and talents, expects to be recognized as superior without commensurate achievements).
2. Is preoccupied with fantasies of unlimited success, power, brilliance, beauty, or ideal love.
3. Believes that he or she is "special" and unique and can only be understood by, or should associate with, other special or high-status people (or institutions).
4. Requires excessive admiration.
5. Has a sense of entitlement (i.e., unreasonable expectations of especially favorable treatment or automatic compliance with his or her expectations).
6. Is interpersonally exploitative (i.e., takes advantage of others to achieve his or her own ends).
7. Lacks empathy: is unwilling to recognize or identify with the feelings and needs of others.
8. Is often envious of others or believes that others are envious of him or her.
9. Shows arrogant, haughty behaviors or attitudes. (American Psychiatric Association, 2013)

Gaslighting in the Workplace

When gaslighting goes undetected within the workplace, persons that have done nothing wrong, can be labeled and lied about by persons who gaslight. Therefore, it is imperative that leadership within organizations be educated on techniques used by bullies and divisive personalities that are disruptive to the work environment. Persons who gaslight are trying to gain control and manipulate another person for personal gain and perceived power. Characteristically, the gaslighter has low self-esteem and self-worth, and there is an attempt to hide their own insecurities by talking negatively about others. Gaslighters are highly manipulative and have difficulty navigating their personal and workplace roles when they feel they are without power. In absence of their ability to psychologically manipulate others, they themselves experience a heightened anxiety of being discovered of how little they may actually know and how disempowered they truly feel. Gaslighters are in fact victims of their own deception as they reside in a world crafted of their own lies.

Heal Thyself

The Cambridge Dictionary defines a *healer* as "a person who has the power to cure ill people without using ordinary medicines: a spiritual healer" and also as "a person or thing that heals: time is a great healer" (Cambridge Dictionary, 2023). Traditionally, nursing has had a historical background of religious and spiritual connections. During the pre-Christian era, the care of the ill was associated with the ability to nourish the souls of others with prayer and was a noble act (Timmins & McSherry, 2012). The embodiment of the spiritual is how nursing was viewed in Celtic ancient writings, and the nurse was referred to as a "soul friend" to the ill to whom they provided care to, or "anam cara" (Grove & Klauser, 2005). Foundationally, nursing is a profession of faith and carries with it the foundational belief that healing is a gift of compassion directed toward others who are in need of nurses' delivery of physical, emotional, and spiritual healing.

Nurses are professional healers. Nurses learn to heal through the recognition of symptomatology associated with different disease processes. However, for nurses when scars turn inward, the nurse as healer experiences emotional wounds that unattended to, manifest as physical and mental illness. To heal thyself is often not possible. Therefore, nurses will require someone to listen, maintaining confidentiality, to their story and situation related to bullying and help them to identify, processes, develop, and plan approaches to heal their pain so that they can move toward action and, ultimately, forgiveness. Because in absence of forgiveness, nurses affected by The Hollow give power to those who bully.

Moving Forward

The purpose of "moving forward" in name, theme, and goal is to inspire others who have encountered bullying and thrived. Mental health, spiritual wellness, and physical heath are protective factors against bullying. When one maintains a work-life balance, they are already proactive in their understanding of the importance of health maintenance and wellness promotion.

The next steps in the acceleration of health and wellness "moving forward" are the following:

1. Acknowledgment that bullying can be an emotional and physical insult to one's body and mind.

2. The spiritual health of persons who are bullied is challenged when the act of harming another mentally and physically is intentionally ignored by others in an attempt to provide an image of unity and belonging.
3. Supporting of plans of change at the micro- and macro-system level in promoting nursing wellness and addressing incivility and bullying within the workplace can easily become stagnant when organizations fear a "reveal" of employees sharing their discontentment with the status quo.
4. Positive change can occur within any work environment. All that is needed is the empowerment of all nursing staff to correct that which is dysfunctional in environments that have historically tolerated bullying and incivility.

Bullying is a painful, often unprovoked act of treating a person unjustly and without cause. For the bully or bullies, they believe that their intentional actions taken to shame, lie, cause doubt, and physically or emotionally harm their targets are warranted because of their own need to self-protect. Bullies view their targets as a potential or actual threat to the exposure of their own deficits. Hence, when exposed by their targets, bullies may attempt to either increase their attack or retreat in fear. The process of the target making the decision to move forward beyond the experience of the bully or bullies is a conscious one that can only be empowered with a counter move to expose the act of incivility and the perpetrators involved.

Summary

Moving forward for the nurse affected by The Hollow is the process of exposing the acts of the bully and making the conscious decision to forgive and resume their own lives before the bully existed. The positive event that occurs post the exposure of the bully or bullies and their acts of incivility is that the affected nurse emerges stronger in character, moral clarity, and an undefeatable resolve. The process of moving forward is one of rebuilding.

Activity

Adult Drawing for Healing and Clarity of Situation

Directions Drawing pictures and coloring can be very relaxing and also thought provoking for adults. When a person draws a picture of how they are feeling, of someone close to them, or a picture of their immediate environment, both consciously and unconsciously, the person(s) is sharing how they are feeling about a particular situation and how they perceive what is occurring. Draw a picture that describes your feelings as you are presently experiencing them now and when recalling an event.

1. Draw a picture of yourself.

2. Draw a part of your body that you are pleased with.

3. Write two words that describe what makes you happy. Draw a picture representing the two words.

4. Draw a picture of your family.

5. Draw a picture of your best friend.

6. Draw a picture of how you feel working as a nurse on a good day.

7. Draw a picture of how you feel working in another role (e.g., mother, wife, son, brother, daughter, etc.).

8. Draw a picture of your face as you prepare to go to work.

9. Draw a picture of your face upon arrival to work.

10. Draw a picture of your face when interacting with patients.

11. Draw a picture of your face and body when interacting with family members.

12. Draw a picture of your face and body when interacting with your co-workers.

13. Draw a picture of yourself if you have ever experienced bullying.

14. Draw a picture of yourself free from the hold of The Hollow.

Activity 47

Upon completion of the drawing activity, consider this:

- After completing your drawings, examine them closely.
- Are you surprised at how your drawings look?
- What do your drawings reveal about you and your current life situation?
- If there is an area in need of improvement, what will be your next steps?
- Identify a person or person (e.g., disclosure to a friend, co-worker, manager, director, spouse, counselor, or therapist) that can help you with you next steps.

Activity

The Act of Moving Forward

The act of moving forward is an exercise in accepting the past and the future to come, as being negotiable. The negotiability is either positive or negative. The decision to no longer be stagnant but to change one's position in life warrants that one be presented with options. With this activity, participants will be asked to "move forward" when they perceive that there is no threat to their safety; physically, emotionally, or spiritually.

Moving Forward Scenarios

1. You are invited to meet with a co-work and another peer. No agenda has been provided. Would you **move forward**?
   Yes or No.
   What is the reason for the rationale you provided?
2. A colleague during a work-related meeting makes a side comment to another colleague about how you handled a situation. What would you do? Should you **move forward** with initiating a conversation about what was said or ignore the conversation as ridiculous and nonsensible?
3. If your story is true, then no one can argue with you about your story not being true. To do the latter means that the person in which you are engaged in a conversation with is lying. What would you do if someone is obviously lying about you in front of others. Do you remain quiet or **move forward** and address the person or persons engaged in the act of lying?
4. To be kind involves being genuine of heart. Knowingly and respectfully acknowledging one's truth or the truth of another. How would you **move forward** knowing that the standard of organizational acceptance is not being kind nor genuine? Should you consider leaving the organization or help promote change by increasing awareness?

References

American Psychiatric Association. (2013). *Diagnostic and statistical manual of mental disorders fifth edition (DSM-5)*. American Psychiatric Publishing.

Boring, R. L. (2020). Implications of narcissistic personality disorder on organizational resilience. In P. Arezes & R. Boring (Eds.), *Advances in safety management and human performance* (AHFE 2020. Advances in intelligent systems and computing) (Vol. 1204, pp. 259–266). Springer. https://link.springer.com/chapter/10.1007/978-3-030-50946-0_35

Cambridge Dictionary. (2023). *Healer*. https://dictionary.cambridge.org/us/dictionary/english/healer

Feilding-Singh, P., & Dmowska, A. (2022). Obstetric gaslighting and the denial of mothers' realities. *Social Science & Medicine, 301*. https://doi.org/10.1016/j.socscimed.2022.114938

Grove, R. F., & Klauser, H. A. (2005). *The American book of the dying: Lessons in healing spiritual pain*. Celestial Arts.

Hamilton, P. (1966). *Angel street: A Victorian thriller in three acts*. Samuel French Inc. Plays.

Johnson, V. E., Nadal, K. L., Gina Sissoko, D. R., & King, R. (2021). "It's not in your head:" Gaslighting, splaining, victim blaming, and other harmful reactions to microaggressions. *Perspectives on Psychological Science: A Journal of the Association of Psychological Science, 16*(5), 1024–1036. https://doi.org/10.1177/17456916211011963

Timmins, F., & McSherry, W. (2012). Spirituality: The holy grail of contemporary nursing practice. *Journal of Nursing Management, 20*(8), 951–957. https://doi.org/10.1111/jonm.12038

Shallow 6

Learning Objectives

1. Explain how the perception of feeling unsupported can impact nurses experiencing The Hollow.
2. Discuss how difficult conversations can facilitate positive change in the work environment.
3. Discuss how continual exposure to work environments that permit incivility can be emotionally and physically damaging to affected nurses.

Shallow

The Merriam-Webster Dictionary (2024) defines the word **shallow** as breathing with minimal depth, moving minimal air in the lungs; lack of knowledge in feelings, thoughts, and depths; reaching only the easily perceived; having little extension backward or inward; and having no depth, such as shallow water. The absence of depth can coincide with risks of harm. For example, diving into shallow water can lead to bodily harm, and shallow breathing can lead to retention of carbon dioxide. And a person who verbally expresses shallow thoughts and feelings usually has no desire to develop a strong bond to those who they are engaging in conversation with or building a relationship. Shallow communication is superficial.

Treading Water

Nurses in the midst of a bullying experience can feel as if they are treading water. Nurse leaders are often reluctant themselves in addressing the bullying. The nurse leader may not want to be perceived by their fellow nurse leaders as aligning with a subordinate. Or the nurse leader may not feel comfortable engaging in what they perceive will be difficult conversations around the bullying the affected nurse is experiencing. As a result, the affected nurse may feel unsupported because they have been intentionally silenced by their manager in attempt to avoid conflict with others involved in the bullying process. Additionally, by silencing the affected nurse, the manager avoids the perception by their director, vice president of nursing, or chief nursing officer, of weakness and an inability to effectively manage their unit and staff.

Difficult Conversations

Difficult conversations occur when a conscious decision is made by two different parties to engage in resolution to an identified problem. Both parties must be willing to maintain honesty and respectfully acknowledge when they are "wrong" and take feedback to correct their actions. Unwillingness to respectfully listen to one another does not bring about healing, nor repair broken lines of communication.

According to Patterson et al. (2012), crucial conversations are necessary when stakes are high. For example, a relationship may be affected, a job loss could occur, a financial transaction may be disrupted, and a business deal upended. Current research supports that when organizations create cultures whereby crucial conversations are embraced, more patient lives are saved within hospitals, financial institutions gain loyal customers and have more financial gains, technology firms can with ease enhance functionalities internationally, and nuclear power plants operate safely (Patterson et al., 2012). Crucial conversations will involve high stakes, opposing opinions, and strong emotions.

When facing crucial conversations, participatory parties may choose to avoid engaging in an open conversation to address the issue(s) at hand, or engage within the conversation but not explore the issues at all. From a positive productivity perspective, participatory parties can decide to face the issues at hand and work toward resolution. The decision to walk away from crucial conversations can be one that may bring regret or inadvertently aid in the maintenance of cultural dysfunction within an organization. The choice is there and awaiting a healthy and empowering decision by each individual.

Hidden Conflict

Shallow motives bring about moments of physical and emotional injury, as the affected nurse attempts to navigate their own perceived truth of the bullying experience while maintaining composure as the bully or bullies decidedly choose to lie. An internal conflict is felt as the belly tightens, heart beats quickly, and the body overheats. Our body reacts to the bully's lies in total disbelief and attempts to reorganize the mind to truly hear and process what has been said. The bully hopes that his or her statements are off putting and uses this strategy as a means to attempt to overpower the other person.

The Maintenance of Truth

The closure to most dilemmas ends with the disclosure of truth. If the person or persons affected by bullying has done nothing wrong, there is no need to exhaust themselves and place their own mental and physical health at risk if they are being lied about. What does it prove? Speak the truth and move forward. It is then up to the organization in which the employees are employed to thoroughly investigate the transaction. If the organization fails to investigate the allegations, and the bullying worsens, it is then that the affected person's health is at greater risk, and an employment lawyer may need to be consulted. The employment attorney should be a last resort. If conflicts, both provoked and unprovoked, can be civilly dealt with within the organizational structure via open and honest communication, it is best to do so. Remember, ultimately, those who have a record of historically distorting the truth will eventually be exposed.

Overexposed

Overexposure to workplaces that ignore bullying can be dangerous to one's health. When bullying is accepted and ignored, organizations leave themselves open to lawsuits. Nurses are more at risk for physical and mental illness development after days, weeks, months, and years of dealing with toxic workplace interactions. Of concern is that organizations are often well aware that there is a problem with bullying but fear having to change a culture. This can be a large undertaking, and to do so requires the organization to admit to its employees that a problem exists.

The public admission of a bullying problem is a brave undertaking which employers believe will leave them legally vulnerable to employees that have had past complaints of experiencing bullying and incivility in the workplace. To the contrary, the admittance of a problem and the resolution to identify and address the problems at hand can also absolve the company of being known for acceptance of "bad" behaviors in the workplace and not responding to employees' complaints. In essence, proof of attempting to absolve the culture of bullying is better than having not tried to at all.

It may bring some comfort to organizations experiencing employee bullying within the workplace that the problem of bullying is international. Germany reports having 17% of their workforce report bullying. In the United States, 30% of the workforce report having experienced bullying; 30% translates to an estimation of 48.6 million working adults. India has an estimated 46% to 55% of workplace bullying (Praslova et al., 2022).

Creating a work environment that not only educates its employees about bullying but discusses the consequences of intentionally physically and mentally harming a fellow employee such as progressive action (verbal and written) discipline that can lead to termination of employment is imperative. Workplaces that demonstrate the valuing of each employee and focus on employee safety are more likely to be healthier places to work. The latter are also workplaces that are less likely to demonize and then ostracize the person reporting having experienced bullying within the organization.

Not an Option

When does the continued acceptance of bullying workplace behaviors become too extreme? Should it be after an employee is openly verbally accosted in front of their fellow employees? Or a physical assault occurs after numerous reports of witnessed verbal bullying and "light shoves" in the hallway while the bully passes by the affected person. When a person or persons submit a notice of resignation to their employer after weeks, months, or years of experiencing workplace bullying? Or, Perhaps it is when an actual suicide has occurred after the person affected by workplace bullying just could not tolerate another day, hour, minute, or second with being bullied. The affected person in the case of a suicide feels helpless and hopeless after being unheard and ignored by their employer and fellow employees (Howard et al., 2021).

The Workplace

Organizational interest in their employees' well-being has historically been a focus because of increased productivity and decrease of turnover intentions. For organizations, in order to maintain a culture whereby bullying is not acceptable behavior and awareness of the effects of bullying, such as depression, gastrointestinal problems, and suicide exists, employers must be openly willing to discuss observations and reports of bullying by employees without judgment. Raycha and Almoula (2023) studied how organizational cultures are impacted when bullying is allowed to remain without intervention. Productivity and profitability are important elements of success for organizations, but neither can occur when employees are allowed to bully their fellow employees. The mission, vision, and values of the organization are shattered as wounded workers infuse the workplace and bullying behaviors are permitted to proliferate. Ultimately, these organizations will encounter financial problems and difficulty in the achievement and sustainability of success within their industries.

Exit, Voice, Loyalty, and Neglect

The Exit, Voice, Loyalty, and Neglect (EVLN) Model (Hirshman, 1970) examines how intent to leave an organization or stay is based upon the organizational culture and how employees take cues from the culture in determining their decisions. Employees who encounter difficult situations (e.g., bullying) within the workplace and desire a change in position may make the decision to either transfer to a different department or resign and **exit** the organization. Some employees may choose to **voice** their concerns to the organization about dissatisfying situations in the workplace like bullying, while others decide that silence is the only option to survive and remain in their current position. Employees' **loyalty** to their organizations ultimately will drive their decision to resign or remain in workplace situations that may be unhealthy. Lastly, the **neglecting** of workplace incidences that are uncivil and result in the continuation of bullying may temporarily lead to employee retention. However, it is the ongoing interface with dysfunctional work environments that will impact productivity and profitability and lead to the decision of employees to decide that in order to maintain physical and mental health, that resignation is their best option.

Summary: Depth

The unknown depth of dark waters can be unnerving. Of concern, is when someone is in dark waters, the depth cannot be determined and drowning can occur. Nurse-to-nurse bullying and incivility are metaphorically representative of dark waters and the unsafe nature of swimming in potentially dangerous waters. Nurses can drown within workplace environments that are isolating and unsupportive.

Activity

Directions Read each workplace scenario. Applying Hirshman's (1970) Exit, Voice, Loyalty, and Neglect (EVLN) Model, select which of the four areas fit the best.

1. Marie felt she had come to a dead end. She had reported her co-worker's argumentative behaviors in staff meetings several times as a concern. Her co-worker consistently sought ways in which she could interrupt or embarrass Marie whenever she spoke during staff meetings. Marie's peers would offer support but only at the end of the meeting, walking quietly in her office and closing the door. The manager and peers all seemed afraid of the bully. Marie made an appointment with her manager and entered the meeting with a resignation letter.
    Question: Which of the four EVLN Model selections best fit Marie's current workplace situation? **Discuss the progression of the situation and the eventual outcome.**
    (a) Exit
    (b) Voice
    (c) Loyalty
    (d) Neglect
2. Bob was angry. He had difficulty hiding his frustration. His face was beet red, and now, his blood pressure had become chronically elevated. Bob was one of those employees who always put his job first and family second. As a senior

administrator at work, he had anticipated that when the position of president became available, his education and vast experience at the company meant that he was the ideal candidate. Bob was deeply hurt when his long-term career goal was disrupted and the company hired a person from outside of the state and requested that Bob train the new President.

Question: Which of the four EVLN Model selections best fit Bob's current workplace situation and his reaction to not being promoted? **Discuss the progression of the situation and the eventual outcome.**
 (a) Exit
 (b) Voice
 (c) Loyalty
 (d) Neglect

3. Sherry was usually silent in team meetings, but when her boss demanded to know if she was up to completing an assignment that she had successfully completed the work for the last 15 years, Sherry was in disbelief. Sherry shared, "I have been at this company for 20 years and worked on this assignment for the last 15 years. I have received numerous awards and accolades for my work. Why am I now being questioned as to my ability to do the work?"

    Question: Which of the four EVLN Model selections best fit Sherry's current workplace situation? **Discuss the progression of the situation and the eventual outcome.**
    (a) Exit
    (b) Voice
    (c) Loyalty
    (d) Neglect

4. Jose frequently communicated his concern that there were problems with a new robotic device used for surgeries in the operating room. The hospital had recently changed vendors. While the cost was substantially lower than the previous vendor, the quality of the product was in question. After communicating his concern to his nurse manager and director, at least six times, Jose became frustrated and decided to say nothing anymore after the nurse manager and director informed him during a meeting that they "Did not appreciate being told (by Jose) how to handle their responsibilities." As a result, Jose isolated himself and chose to use silence as a means to cope with being unheard and, in his perception, disrespected. Three months after the new robotic device was introduced, the device malfunctioned during a procedure causing significant burns to a patient and nurse.

    Jose decided to report his prior complaints to his nurse manager and director to the chief nursing officer and vice president of operations. After his report, he received minimal communication or support. Jose then documented his concerns and shared them with the Department of Public Health (DPH) and the Occupational Safety and Health Administration (OSHA). An investigation is currently in process regarding Jose's shared concerns about device safety.

    Question: Which of the four EVLN Model selections best fit Jose's current workplace situation? **Discuss the progression of the situation and the eventual outcome.**

(a) Exit
(b) Voice
(c) Loyalty
(d) Neglect

Answers

Question 1: (a); Exit
Question 2: (g); Loyalty
Question 3: (j); Voice
Question 4: (d); Neglect

Activity

Depth or No Depth: Shallow

Directions Read each statement and identify whether the statement has depth or no depth (is shallow). Circle depth or no depth after each statement.

1. **Circle Depth or No Depth.** "I am not sure just how smart she really is, but I do know that I have a lot more know how."
2. **Circle Depth or No Depth.** "I like to listen to him. He offers wisdom and insight."
3. **Circle Depth or No Depth.** "We can solve this problem together."
4. **Circle Depth or No Depth.** "We should pull together and see if we can take over the situation. Autonomy is not needed in this situation. Who cares about what they think."
5. **Circle Depth or No Depth.** "If we work as a team, we can succeed together."

References

Hirschman, A. O. (1970). *Exit, voice, and loyalty: Responses to decline in firms, organizations, and states.* Harvard University Press.

Howard, M. C., Follmer, K. B., Smith, M. B., Tucker, R. P., & Van Zandt, E. C. (2021). Work and suicide: An interdisciplinary systematic literature review. *Journal of Organizational Behavior, 43*(2), 260–285. https://doi.org/10.1002/job.2519

Merriam-Webster Dictionary. (2024). *Shallow.* https://www.merriam-webster.com/dictionary/shallow

Patterson, K., Grenny, J., McMillan, R., & Switzler, A. (2012). *Crucial conversations: Tools for talking when stakes are high.* McGraw Hill.

Praslova, L. N., Carucci, R., & Stokes, C. (2022). How bullying manifests at work—And how to stop it. *Harvard Business Review*. https://hbr.org/2022/11/how-bullying-manifests-at-work-and-how-to-stop-it

Raycha, B. P., & Almoula, T. S. (2023). Sustaining organizational culture amid workplace bullying: A review of employee responses using EVLN model. *IUP Journal of Organizational Behavior, 22*(3), 87–109.

The Depths of Forgetfulness 7

Learning Objectives

1. Explain how forgetting when wronged by someone can be difficult.
2. Discuss the necessity of forgiveness in moving beyond experiences of workplace bullying and incivility.
3. Discuss how continual exposure to work environments that permit the emergence of symptomatology surrounding The Hollow can impact affected nurses psychologically and physically.

Forgetfulness

Forgetfulness is the state of being unable to recall an event. Forgetfulness warrants that something that was to be remembered is not easily recalled. However, the pain and recall of a traumatic event provide an opportunity for those who were hurt to remember, reflect, and heal.

The Merriam -Webster Dictionary defines the word **forgetfulness** as inducing oblivion (forgetful sleep), being likely to be forgetful, and the characterization of being neglectful related to a failure to remember (Merriam-Webster Dictionary, 2024). The complexity of the word forgetfulness materializes in the discussion of The Hollow Theory because when someone experiences physical harm or emotional abuse, it is the mental replay (Green, 2019) of the actual incident of bullying and incivility that paralyzes them. The repetition of the traumatizing memory can become incapacitating affecting sleep, appetite, the ability to concentrate, and trust and engagement with others.

© The Author(s), under exclusive license to Springer Nature
Switzerland AG 2025
C. Green, *How Can Nurses Survive Bullying Environments?*,
https://doi.org/10.1007/978-3-031-86617-3_7

Forgiveness

Forgiveness is the only means by which the mental replay of the traumatizing event can be redefined in the mind of persons affected by The Hollow. While the ability for a human being to forget traumatic events may not always occur, the pain generated from emotionally laden experiences can cause persons with The Hollow, to feel empty, unloved, not cared for, and isolated. These false narratives unaddressed by counseling and support both inside and outside the work environment, can lead to disturbances in mental health.

The American Psychological Association (APA) defines **forgiveness** as the decision to willfully put aside resentment toward someone who has been hurtful, harmed you, been unfair, or wronged you (APA, 2024). The act of forgiveness is transformative. In order to fully forgive another person that has harmed you, resentment is no longer the focus nor is anger. The person who forgives exhibits generosity and compassion toward the person who harmed them (APA, 2024). While not easily obtained, forgiveness releases the wronged person from the restrictive bondage of anger and hatred toward the person that harmed them and allows them to move forward in their lives toward happiness and positive productivity.

From a scriptural perspective, the forgiveness of others is healing. Below are some scriptural references about forgiving others (Holy Bible, New International Version, 1984).

2 Corinthians 2: 7–8. Now, instead, you ought to forgive and comfort him, so that he will not be overwhelmed by excessive sorrow. I urge you, therefore, to reaffirm your love for him.
Matthew 6:12. Forgive us our debts, as we also have forgiven our debtors.
Ephesians 4:31–32. Get rid of all bitterness, rage and anger, brawling and slander, along with every form of malice. Be kind and compassionate to one another, forgiving each other, just as in Christ God forgive you.
Luke 17: 3–4 If your brother sins, rebuke him, and if he repents, forgive him. If he sins against you seven times in a day, and seven times comes back to you and says, "I repent, forgive him."
Matthew 6:14–15. If you forgive men when they sin against you, your heavenly Father will also forgive you. But if you do not forgive men their sins, your Father will not forgive your sins.

Being bullied is difficult. The affected person feels that they have literally loss control of their own lives and the outcome of their future selves. However, the latter is a lie of which the bully or bullies wish to bestow or feed to the mind of the person(s) they are bulling to gain control. Power is a perception only, and not all perceptions are based on reality. For the person experiencing The Hollow, forgiveness can be their greatest asset in terms of self-protection against incivility and bullying. Rationally, the conscious decision to forgive persons who have wronged you releases you from their perceived power to enter a new journey and adventure in your life whereby the wrong behaviors that were used against you are subdued and rendered useless. You are free!

The Danger of Workplace Bullying

Workplace bullying is dangerous to affected persons because the emotionally injured person is not within a silo. The bullied person leaves work and returns to a family, friendships, church, marriages, intimate relationships, other jobs, and activities of daily living (e.g., going to the bank or grocery shopping). Hence, the bullied person reciprocally interacts with society and the organization in which the bullying is occurring (Tuckey & Neall, 2014). **Emotional injury** occurs when someone has been repeatedly attacked verbally and either withdraws or projects their suppressed feelings on others in their immediate environments and within random encounters. Emotionally injured persons may verbally abuse others or could potentially physically harm another, as suppressed anger, hostility, and a perceived need to protect oneself from bullying, envelopes the affected person.

For nurses working within healthcare organizations, the immediate environment constitutes the healthcare environment and the patients to whom they are providing nursing care. Because the patient is the primary focus of nurses in their work within healthcare organizations, it is the patient(s) that can become the unintended target of the bullied nurses' emotional injury. Therefore, verbal abuse, being ignored, speaking abruptly and walking away, and making medication or treatment errors may occur to patients being cared for by bullied nurses.

According to Johnson and Benham-Hutchins (2020), nursing errors are more likely to occur within the context of bullying. Arnetz et al. (2020) found that nurse work environments that were associated with poor nurse health and bullying could result in adverse patient events (e.g., central-line associated bloodstream infections). Therefore, workplaces that permit or choose to ignore occurrences and reports of bullying may have more errors impacting patients. It is important to note that nursing teams where bullying is allowed will likely have impaired communication barriers amongst team members because the team consists of nurses who bully and nurses who are recipients of their uncivil conduct.

Quiet Quitting

Quiet Quitting occurs when an employee who is dissatisfied with their employer begins to gradually reduce their work productivity and overall performance, rather than submitting a resignation letter. During the coronavirus 2019 (COVID-19) pandemic, employees took to social media platforms such as TikTok to share how they were quietly quitting their jobs (Harter, 2023; Lord, 2022; Scheyett, 2022). Debatably, quiet quitting is believed not to be a new phenomenon, but one that has been practiced in industry for several years (Lord, 2022). Harter (2023), upon review of US Gallup noted that it is estimated that at least 50% of workers make up "quiet quitters." Engaged workers make up (Harter, 2023) 32% with 18% of employees actively disengaging. In healthcare settings, studies on quiet quitting have found that over 50% of healthcare employees engage in quiet quitting (Galanis et al., 2023, 2024a).

Nurses who experience The Hollow have experienced bullying. Bullying is a type of workplace violence. Nurses subjected to bullying, unless provided support at the unit level from peers and managers, will likely leave their jobs. Experiencing post-traumatic stress disorder (PTSD), physical health problems, stress, anxiety, decrease in work productivity and work quality, depression, burnout, low self-esteem, and job dissatisfaction, nurses' turnover intentions increase (Al Muharraq et al., 2022; Galanis et al., 2024b; Goh et al., 2022; Karatuna et al., 2020). Younger and older nurses are impacted by bullying. However, it is often the newer nurse that receives the unhealthy initiation of bullying and dysfunctional behaviors associated with bullying (Anusiewicz et al., 2019; Karatuna et al., 2020) from the experienced nurse(s).

Wronged

There is a sense, a feeling of having been wronged when bullying occurs in the workplace. The intent of the bully or bullies is to set the other person(s) up to be harmed in some way. Bullies may use attacks of character, lying, and sabotaging of one's work, all underhanded attempts at casting the affected person in a shadow of being questionably a troublemaker. When a person experiences The Hollow at work and at home in their personal life, the duality of the stress and simultaneous abuse warrants immediate therapeutic intervention. Bitterness, anger, frustration, and distrust (Lutzer, 2007) can envelope the affected person and will eventually impede their personal and professional lives. In this case, professional counseling should be sought in order for distinct patterns of behavioral reactions to bullies and the action of bullying to be addressed successfully. Sometimes insight into why one allows certain personality types and behavioral patterns to persist in their lives can bring resolution to the bullying problem as the affected person recognizes unhealthy people in their lives and begins to set boundaries regarding what they will and will not tolerate.

Summary: Unearthing Forgetfulness

In order for healthcare organizations to end bullying and retain nurses, training must be initiated at the staff level all the way up to managerial, administrative, and senior level leadership on the dangers of ignoring bullying. Current research (and articles) on workplace bullying has shown that patients' health outcomes are impacted and affected nurses' mental and physical health, and nurse suicide (Ahc Media, 2020; Mental Health Practice, 2018) can occur as a result of prolonged exposure to toxic workplaces. While organizations would like to forget that bullying has occurred because acknowledgment of bullying behaviors is viewed as bad publicity, the bullied nurse suffers alone in isolation and their patients are unintentionally harmed.

Putting Forgiveness into Practice

A Personal Activity

Directions Forgiveness is a process. Sometimes in relationships, only one party forgives the other. And, sometimes, forgiveness can occur between two or more persons, resulting in peace and complete resolution of the problem. In the latter case, persons can walk away without bitterness. It is important to remember that forgiveness is an individual process that allows those impacted by negative situations, to positively move forward in absence of the burden of unforgiveness. In this activity, select and discuss a personal action that involves forgiveness. Consider how your personal reaction may impact the situation.

Personal Activity #1
A co-worker constantly interrupts you during meetings when you are contributing to a group discussion. Does this warrant a one-to-one conversation, or should the co-worker's behavior be dismissed and forgiven?

Personal Activity #2
A manager steals your ideas and presents them as their own during a corporate presentation. Taken aback, you feel hurt and betrayed and decide to leave the meeting early. As you return to your office, your manager requests you to return to the meeting immediately because they would like one of your ideas "explained in more detail to the team." You pause and decide to return to the meeting. The manager acknowledges your presence and kindly asks you to share your ideas.

Did this manager betray you? Are the manager's actions forgivable?

Personal Activity #3
You are at a corporate compliance training event with colleagues. The lead trainer provides the opportunity for participants to take a 50-min break to eat their lunch. During lunch, two co-workers from another department sit at the table that you have already begun to eat lunch at with two other colleagues. As a friendly conversation ensues, one of the colleagues from a different department states directly to you, "You are really nice. You are nothing like we heard you were." Unsure as to what this meant, you continue to eat your lunch quietly. Should you address this comment after the training event? Ignore the comment? Or inquire, why the comment was asked and who shared that you were difficult to communicate with?

Personal Activity #4

Loneliness is isolating, makes a person feel depressed, and have a yearning to belong. As a young biracial executive who practices Judaism, I have openly experienced discrimination within the workplace. My director is aware and has said very little to my co-workers, or supported me. It has been 1 year since my employment in my current position. I am not quite certain how to address my co-workers' and director's intentional disregard for discrimination in the workplace. Should I report what is happening to Human Resources or the Vice President of the division? Or, both?

Personal Activity #5

The bullying has impacted my life negatively, more than I care to admit. Most days I do not want to go to work. I feel alone, sad, detached, and cry most of the work day intermittently. I am not certain what my next steps should be because I have been working in this environment for 8 years, and it appears to only be getting worse. My personality has changed. I am not as confident as I use to be and I know it. I need to make a change, but I am not certain of what my next steps should be and where I should go after so many years working at the same company. What should I do? How should I proceed?

Personal Activity #6

Lately, I have been just thinking about ending my life. I have gone to Human Resources and spoken numerous times with my manager and director, and nothing has improved in my work situation. The bullying has worsened. Sometimes I wake up and dread going to work. I argue with family members over very simple things and isolate myself when I am at work. I am starting to have thoughts of just ending it all. I am just not happy with my life. What should I do? Should I talk to someone? What should be my next steps?

References

Ahc Media. (2020). Research on nurses' suicide risk reveals ethical concerns. *Medical Ethics Advisor, 36*(2), N.PAG.

Al Muharraq, E. H., Baker, O. G., & Alallah, S. M. (2022). The prevalence and the relationship of workplace bullying and nurses' turnover intentions: A cross sectional study. *SAGE Open Nursing, 24*(8), 23779608221074655. https://doi.org/10.1177/23779608221074655

American Psychological Association (APA). (2024). *Forgiveness*. https://www.apa.org/topics/forgiveness

Anusiewicz, C. V., Shirey, M. R., & Patrician, P. A. (2019). Workplace bullying and newly licensed registered nurses: An evolutionary concept analysis. *Workplace Health & Safety, 67*(5), 250–261. https://doi.org/10.1177/2165079919827046

Arnetz, J. E., Neufcourt, L., Sudan, S., Arnetz, B. B., Maiti, T., & Viens, F. (2020). Nurse-reported bullying and documented adverse patient events: An exploratory study in a US hospital. *Journal of Nursing Care Quality, 35*(3), 206–212. https://doi.org/10.1097/ncq.0000000000000442

References

Galanis, P., Katsiroumpa, A., Vraka, I., Siskou, O., Konstantakopoulou, O., Katsoulas, T., Moisoglou, I., Gallos, P., & Kaitelidou, D. (2023). *The influence of job burnout on quiet quitting among nurses: The mediating effect of job satisfaction.* https://www.researchgate.net/publication/372094983_The_influence_of_job_burnout_on_quiet_quitting_among_nurses_the_mediating_effect_of_job_satisfaction

Galanis, P., Moisoglou, I., Malliarou, M., Papathanasiou, I. V., Katsiroumpa, A., Vraka, I., Siskou, O., Konstantakopoulou, O., & Kaitelidou, D. (2024a). Quiet quitting among nurses increases their turnover intention: Evidence from Greece in the post-COVID-19 era. *Healthcare, 12*(1), 79. https://doi.org/10.3390/healthcare12010079

Galanis, P., Moisoglou, I., Katsiroumpa, A., & Mastrogianni, M. (2024b). Association between workplace bullying, job stress, and professional quality of life in nurses: A systematic review and meta-analysis. *Healthcare (Basel), 12*(6), 623. https://doi.org/10.3390/healthcare12060623

Goh, H. S., Hosier, S., & Zhang, H. (2022). Prevalence, antecedents, and consequences of workplace bullying among nurses – A summary of reviews. *International Journal of Environmental Research & Public Health, 19*(14), 8256. https://doi.org/10.3390/ijerph19148256

Green, C. (2019). *Incivility among nursing professionals in clinical and academic environments: Emerging research and opportunities.* IGI Global.

Harter, J. (2023). Is quiet quitting real? *Workplace.* https://www.gallup.com/workplace/398306/quiet-quitting-real.aspx

International Bible Society. (1984). *Holy bible* (New International Version). Zondervan Publishing House.

Johnson, A. H., & Benham-Hutchins, M. (2020). The influence of bullying on nursing practice errors: A systematic review. *Association of Perioperative Registered Nurses Journal, 111*(2), 199–210. https://doi.org/10.1002/aorn.12923

Karatuna, I., Jönsson, S., & Muhonen, T. (2020). Workplace bullying in the nursing profession: A cross-cultural scoping review. *International Journal of Nursing Studies, 111*, 103628. https://doi.org/10.1016/j.ijnurstu.2020.103628

Lord, J. (2022). Quiet quitting is a new name for an old method of industrial action. *The Conversation.* https://www.researchgate.net/publication/363415148_Quiet_quitting_is_a_new_name_for_an_old_method_of_industrial_action

Lutzer, E. W. (2007). *When you've been wronged: Moving from bitterness to forgiveness.* Moody Publishers.

Merriam-Webster Dictionary. (2024). *Forgetful.* https://www.merriam-webster.com/dictionary/forgetfulness

Nurse took her own life after being "bullied" at work. (2018). *Mental Health Practice, 21*(9), 6. https://doi-org.acu.idm.oclc.org/10.7748/mhp.21.9.6.s3

Scheyett, A. (2022). Quiet quitting. *Social Work, 68*, 5–7. https://doi.org/10.1093/sw/swac051

Tuckey, M. R., & Neall, A. M. (2014). Workplace bullying erodes job and personal resources: Between- and within-person perspectives. *Journal of Occupational Health Psychology, 19*(4), 413–424. https://doi.org/10.1037/a0037728

The Depths of Regret 8

Learning Objectives

1. Explain how regret negatively impacts the bullied nurse who decides not to report their workplace experience with incivility targeted at them.
2. Discuss the implications of regret for onlookers of nurse bullying—further violence or nurse suicide.
3. Consider how a reset can positively impact a regret.

Regret Defined

Regret is defined by the Merriam-Webster Dictionary as both a noun and verb. Regret defined as a verb is to be very sorry for mistakes made, to experience a regret, to mourn the death or loss of someone or something, and to miss very much. The word regret used as a noun recognizes a distressing emotion such as a sorrow or a deep sorrow that was aroused by life circumstances that were beyond the affected person's power or control to repair (Merriam-Webster Dictionary Online, 2024). Regret can bring to affected persons, loneliness, frustration, and sadness.

The Hollow

For nurses who experience The Hollow in the workplace, the perception that their being mobbed by co-workers in a meeting, a co-worker is attempting to belittle their skills or perpetuate lies, is not serious enough to report to managers, directors, or Human Resources Department. The nurses' concern may be that there is no proof of bullying. A later report of these incidences in the setting of the bully or bullies presenting with a significant lie leading to an attack on character of the affected nurse is then considered a new investigation of a first act of uncivil conduct. Hence, though difficult, it is important that someone is made aware of these acts of incivility by the affected nurse (or someone who has witnessed the incident such as a co-worker), the first time these behaviors present as an issue.

The Targets

Bullies target nurses who tend to be focused on their jobs, have potential for promotion, introduce cultural innovation or change, are culturally (e.g., religion, linguistics, etc.) and racially different, show no interest in joining their clicks, and present as free thinkers. Bullies tend to be stagnant in their approach to change and prefer to maintain the status quo. Typically, underperformer bullies target those who they perceive may threaten their (the bully's) personal or professional success(es) by exposing who they really are and the knowledge they have or do not have. While the target may not understand this and only sees the meanness, lies, and covert actions of the bully or bullies at work, many bullies are very insecure people who hide behind a pompous personality façade.

Targets tend to suffer from imposter syndrome. **Imposter syndrome** occurs when, persons, despite their intellectual accomplishments (e.g., education level attainment, career success, etc.) and personal and professional successes, feel undeserving and that their successes may have occurred for other reasons outside of their own work and determination. Nursing is a profession that involves emotional and physical connectiveness to patients (families and significant others) that are known for very short or long periods of time by the nurse. Hence, because nurses are providing healthcare to others, a level of vulnerability occurs, whether the nurse positively or negatively connects with patients in their care. For nurses, their care of patients and their loved ones on a routine basis can contribute to the development of burnout, compassion satisfaction, or compassion fatigue (Cetrano et al., 2017; Clark et al., 2022).

The vulnerability of the nurse experiencing The Hollow, because of being targeted by a bully or bullies, can cause nurses to consider leaving the profession of nursing and or resigning from their job. Needless to say, becoming the target of another when striving to maintain health and well-being in the workplace is fatiguing. However, consequentially, bullying, reframed, is a workplace occurrence that is a nuisance. And that which is a nuisance is an annoyance that may or may not cause a person harm. It is the decision to approach bullying as illogical foolishness that is a waste of time and emotional and physical energy that can help affected persons survive incidences of bullying.

The Broken Bully

Persons who bully are usually psychologically vulnerable themselves. Negative childhood events or early adulthood trauma may lead to persons who bully being angry, saddened, and lacking trust. Their psychological vulnerability becomes a defense mechanism that causes them to strike out at others not to protect themselves but to relive their own fantasies of vengeance on those that hurt them in the past. Bullies' trauma is often cyclic and has nothing to do with their current situation. It is the bully's anger, sadness, and lack of trust that causes them to distort seemingly harmless interactions and perceive them as threat. An example of a scenario demonstrating the overreaction of the bully is provided below.

Scenario 1: Bully Overreaction

Richard hated to be questioned about any decision he made. He had been a nurse manager for 8 years and felt that he had more than enough experience to manage the two units that he oversaw for the last 2 years. Michael, a nurse manager for 23 years of four units noticed that Richard had a significant turnover of nursing staff on his two units occurring over the last 3 months. Michael offered to help Richard investigate why his nursing staff was leaving his units. Richard shared, "Michael, I am here to support and mentor you whenever you need me. I was a young manager once myself."

Richard was angry and offended that Michael would have the audacity to question his ability to manage his own unit. Thereafter, Richard would gossip and spread negative lies about Michael without reason. Richard's own insecurities about being perceived as an ineffective manager drove him to undermine a colleague who had merely offered to help him investigate the cause of his nursing staff's turnover intentions.

Insecurities in the person or persons who bully other people lead to their own demise because they ensnare themselves in the imaginary world they create in order to justify their deception. For persons experiencing The Hollow, understanding that the person who bullies is actually weak and vulnerable themselves helps to bring awareness to the frivolousness of the actions of others that have to basis in the truth. The bully shares their own manufactured distortions about how they want others to perceive you.

The Emotional Voice

The emotional voice (EV) is either a voice of reason and sound rationale or of confusion and intentionally remiss of truth versus evil. Be it the voice of a co-worker, boss, supervisor, president, chief officer, manager, a family member, close friend, spouse, or significant other, the speech with emotional expressions and vocalizations (Pell et al., 2022) brings context to the communication being shared between people. For example, if a person is raising the tone of their voice and crying uncontrollably, they may be perceived as being weak and vulnerable by onlookers. The face of the crying person is sad and remorseful and can appear indecisive.

Within the context of bullying and persons experiencing The Hollow, the person who bullies will use their observation of EV to determine how, when, and what words and situations they can use to manipulate the person or persons they are targeting. According to Giordano et al. (2021), affective science theories have examined continuous dimensional attributes such as negative vocal emotions and intense vocalizations and perceptions of emotional stimuli such as a voice that sounds angry. Perceptions of emotions are not always based on reality. Emotional perceptions observed or heard by different persons may produce varied thoughts of personal threat—harm to self or harm to others.

An example of the perception of the emotional voice as angry has been linked to different people groups. For example, some ethnic groups have been perceived to be louder or more emotional than others (Cowen et al., 2019). The angry Black woman or the loud Italian. While these perceptions are not 100% accurate, they breed racism and misunderstanding. While, acoustically, there are some variations among different people from varied cultural backgrounds, this does not account for individual personalities and life experiences.

Regret in the Workplace: Why Is This Unhealthy Behavior Tolerated Anyway

Unhealthy workplaces are unfortunately a common occurrence. A workplace survey taken by the American Psychological Association entitled *2024 Work in America Survey*, noted that 59% of employees think that their employers believe their workplace to be healthier than it actually is in reality. The APA survey found that 39% of employees believe that if they shared with their employer that they were experiencing a mental health condition, this would not have a positive impact on their career.

Resignations can occur in the workplace for a variety of reasons including that of employee relocation, corporate restructuring, job instability, promotion to a higher-level position, or general unhappiness with the type of work the employee is doing. Sull et al. (2022) in an article written within the Massachusetts Institute of Technology (MIT) Sloan Management Review implemented research that investigated why people leave their jobs and analyzed over 170 organizational cultural issues that can impact employee attrition. Sull et al.'s (2022) research occurred during the months of April through September 2021, during the global pandemic of the coronavirus 2019 (COVID-19). Culture 500 companies were included in the study. Culture 500 companies are companies that excel in these nine areas: performance, innovation, respect, integrity, customer orientation, agility, diversity, and collaboration (Sull & Sull, 2020). The five top predictors of attrition identified were:

Poor response to COVID-19: 1.8
Failure to recognize employee performance: 2.9
High levels of innovation: 3.2
Job insecurity and reorganization: 3.5
Toxic corporate culture: 10.4

Interestingly, despite having otherwise healthy cultures, these top-performing Culture 500 companies shared in common the existence of toxic corporate cultures. Hence, toxic work environments can exist anywhere and are by no means a reflection of company failure. Instead, companies can take the approach of maintaining or establishing healthy work environments, by acknowledging the need for their existence and then actively and unashamedly, pursuing change.

Navigating Workplace Change in Real Time

Work cultures are complex and not easily changed. On average, it can take 3–5 years to change a workplace culture. Within the profession of nursing, healthy workplace cultures are imperative for the maintenance of patient safety in healthcare environments. Classically, the view that a *just culture* can contribute to increased patient safety in healthcare promotes the ideology of systems thinking. In just *cultures*, emphasis is placed on the systems' failures to address dysfunction and promote healthy and sustained organizational change, rather than the errors of individuals working within the system (Alashram et al., 2024). While the latter is true and applicable to nurse bullying if the system has intentionally ignored malfunctioning unit cultures for years that have bullying problems, the responsibility must also be placed on the bullies themselves as well.

The allowance of The Hollow to remain active on known clinical units and in departments within healthcare organizations is often a failure of systems to openly address incivility and take a stance for zero tolerance of workplace bullying. Imboden (2024) explored the value and health benefits of people having a sense of belonging in organizations. Belonging is an essential human need in order to function in social situations. Absence of connectivity to others leads to isolation, impacts well-being and trust, and affects employees' health (Imboden, 2024).

In order to change workplace cultures, systems have to change. In order for systems to change, administration has to acknowledge problems that exist within their organization. In order for problems to be discovered, directors and managers have to ask for and receive openly the feedback from their direct patient care staff. For nurses, united, they must reach out for support to one another and to their American Nurses Association so that they have a clear understanding of the Code of Ethics for Nurses (American Nurses Association, n.d.) and how these codes apply to their daily nursing practice.

Nurses must realize that they have the unique gift as healthcare professionals working directly with patients and spending the greatest amount of direct clinical practice hours with patients daily and are best positioned to promote organizational change. No longer can bedside nurse leaders say, "I am just the nurse." Know that your critical thinking and clinical judgment saves the lives of human beings that you interface with as you practice each day you enter the workplace. You have more power than you think. Discover your power, own it, share it, and do not let others attempt to take what is yours on their terms.

Activity

Change

Directions Read each scenario and identify if change is needed in the workplace. Write down the steps you would take to make this change happen.

Scenario #1
A new night nurse is abrupt and curses at her co-workers when they are not "immediately" ready to provide handoff report to so she can "go home."

Is change needed?

Why is change needed?

How can you make this change happen?

Scenario #2
A manager announces that they have selected two nurses to attend a research conference to represent the hospital.

Is change needed?

Why is change needed?

How can you make this change happen?

Scenario #3
A director announces that nurses on a 40-bed medical-surgical unit will be penalized via a new point system if they do not take their required 30-min break each time they work. A cumulation of a total of five points will lead to a negative write up related to the affected nurses poor time management. The unit is currently hiring for six full-time registered nurse positions.

Is change needed?

Why is change needed?

How can you make this change happen?

Scenario #4
A nurse observes one of her nurse colleagues being screamed at by a fellow co-worker. The altercation occurs outside of a patient's hospital room.

Is change needed?

Why is change needed?

How can you make this change happen?

Scenario #5
A patient throws a picture of water on a Latino nurse. The patient yells, "Go back to your country and take care of people that look like you, not me!"

Is change needed?

Why is change needed?

How can you make this change happen?

Scenario #6
A nurse manager informs an African American nurse that she "may not fit in" on the new hospital campus that she has transferred to and recommends she returns to her former "inner city hospital."

Is change needed?

Why is change needed?

How can you make this change happen?

Scenario #7
A nurse is walking into the hospital garage when he is approached by three other nurses. The nurses begin to push and shove the nurse. One of the three nurses proceeds to spit in the nurse's face. You are sitting in your car preparing to leave work when you observe this situation.

Consider this:

Is the nurse in a safe situation?

Is the nurse able to safely leave the situation.

Is change needed?

Why is change needed?

How can you make this change happen?

Scenario #8
A nurse receives an award for providing life-saving care to a fellow hospital employee in the parking lot.

Is change needed?

Why is change needed?

How can you make this change happen?

Scenario #9
Two nurses have been known bullies on a unit for the past 8 years. A newly hired nurse observes these nurses' bullying behaviors and immediately reports them to the manager and Human Resources. The new nurse is now being bullied each time she enters the workplace. The nurse has become depressed and withdrawn.

Is change needed?

Why is change needed?

How can you make this change happen?

Scenario #10
A nurse confides in you that as a result of being bullied for 9 months, she has recently contemplated suicide.

Is change needed?

Why is change needed?

How can you make this change happen?

A Contemplation Activity

Regret

Directions Read each statement or question and discuss how regret likely impacted the outcome.

1. A nurse informs their nurse manager that they are resigning from their career of 20 years sharing, "I just cannot take this toxic environment anymore." The nurse is 2 months away from retirement.
2. A manager is hospitalized after a severe emotional break following an argument with her director. The manager's director had been sarcastic and belittling to him for the last 4 years.
3. Lonely, a nurse contemplates self-harm after an incident of bullying with a night shift nurse. A co-worker observes the nurse taking pills out of her locker and quietly placing them in a small plastic bag. The co-worker stops the nurse and asks if everything is o.k.
4. A nursing professor presenting a research project to a group of colleagues is questioned harshly post presentation as to the credibility of the research findings. The professor leaves the room in silence and returns to their office, closes the door, and cries.
5. A nurse, after being bullied on their clinical unit for 9 months, obtains the new position of unit educator. Very much aware of the bullying problem on the unit, the nurse initiates a series of lectures and activities on the unit that address bullying and the consequences for retaliation.

References

Alashram, H. M., Hamouda, G. M., & Yaseen, M. (2024). Nurses' perception toward the relationship between just culture and patient safety activities: A literature review. *Journal of Health, Medicine & Nursing, 10*(2), 18–33. https://doi-org.acu.idm.oclc.org/10.47604/jhmn.2499

American Nurses Association. (n.d.). *View the Code of Ethics for nurses*. https://www.nursingworld.org/practice-policy/nursing-excellence/ethics/code-of-ethics-for-nurses/

American Psychological Association. (2024). *2024 Work in America Survey: Psychological safety in the changing workplace*. https://www.apa.org/pubs/reports/work-in-america/2024/2024-work-in-america-report.pdf

Cetrano, G., Tedeschi, F., Rabbi, L., Gosetti, G., Lora, A., Lamonaca, D., Manthorpe, J., & Amaddeo, F. (2017). How are compassion fatigue, burnout, and compassion satisfaction affected by quality of working life? Findings from a survey of mental health staff in Italy. *BMC Health Services Research, 17*(1), 755. https://doi.org/10.1186/s12913-017-2726-x

Clark, P., Holden, C., Russell, M., & Downs, H. (2022). The impostor phenomenon in mental health professionals: Relationships among compassion fatigue, burnout, and compassion satisfaction. *Contemporary Family Therapy, 44*(2), 185–197. https://doi.org/10.1007/s10591-021-09580-y

Cowen, A. S., Laukka, P., Elfenbein, H. A., Liu, R., & Keltner, D. (2019). The primacy of categories in the recognition of 12 emotions in speech prosody across two cultures. *Nature Human Behavior, 3*(4), 369–382. https://doi.org/10.1038/s41562-019-0533-6

Giordano, B. L., Whiting, C., Kriegeskorte, N., Kotz, S. A., Gross, J., & Belin, P. (2021). The representational dynamics of perceived voice emotions evolve from categories to dimensions. *Nature Human Behavior, 5*(9), 1203–1213. https://doi.org/10.1038/s41562-021-01073-0

Imboden, M. T. (2024). Belonging: An essential human and organizational need. *American Journal of Health Promotion, 38*(6), 883–897. https://doi-org.acu.idm.oclc.org/10.1177/08901171241255204

Merriam-Webster Dictionary. (2024). *Regret*. https://www.merriam-webster.com/dictionary/regret

Pell, M. D., Sethi, S., Rigoulot, S., Rothermich, K., Liu, P., & Jiang, X. (2022). Emotional voices modulate perception and predictions about an upcoming face. *Cortex, 149*, 148–164. https://doi.org/10.1016/j.cortex.2021.12.017

Sull, D., & Sull, C. (2020, October 13). Cultural excellence. *MIT Sloan Management Review*. https://sloanreview.mit.edu/projects/culture-500-introducing-the-2020-culture-champions/

Sull, D., Sull, C., & Zweig, B. (2022, January 11). Toxic culture is driving the greatest resignation. *MIT Sloan Management Review*. https://sloanreview.mit.edu/article/toxic-culture-is-driving-the-great-resignation/

Simplifying Life

9

Learning Objectives

1. Consider how simplifying one's life can benefit their overall health and well-being.
2. Discuss the implications of not prioritizing work-life balance within the context of experiencing workplace bullying.
3. Learning the importance of rest is important to restorative sleep, relaxation, and renewal of energy.

Work-Life Balance

To maintain a **work-life balance is to ensure that your work and home life seldom intermingle**. For example, a work-related problem may be discussed within the home or within a personal situation with a friend or colleague, but the problem is not the predominant factor nor focus. When work-life balance is managed, care of one's self is prioritized, health and well-being is important, and time and energy is balanced. Often, it is when a person does not balance their time and energy toward their home life being one of contentment that toxic work environments can strangulate the mind and body causing mental fatigue and physical strain (Gragnano et al., 2020).

An unhealthy work-life balance, according to Cook-Campbell (2023) includes burnout, constant overwork, lack of self-care, strained relationships, and neglected personal life. Persons who overwork, tend to have higher incidences of physical illness and depression and anxiety (el Batawi, 1984; Kivimäki et al., 2015; Virtanen et al., 2011). Symptomatology suggestive of a poor work-life balance according to Cook-Campbell (2023) is lack of energy, constantly thinking about work, unexplained aches and pains, restlessness when not at work, struggling to take time off

© The Author(s), under exclusive license to Springer Nature
Switzerland AG 2025
C. Green, *How Can Nurses Survive Bullying Environments?*,
https://doi.org/10.1007/978-3-031-86617-3_9

or a vacation, and money that is spent trying to outsource home chores (e.g., laundry, house cleaning, etc.) due to lack of time at home.

Simplifying Life

The **simplification of one's life involves the recognition of the brevity of life and that the circumstantiality of negative behaviors and outcomes persist for a season only**. In other words, change, no matter how difficult the situation, can occur. It is the realization that it is the moment-to-moment glimpses of peace and tranquility that can bring about hope for the future.

Below are ten tips for simplifying one's life:

1. Kiss a person you love each day and tell them you appreciate them.
2. Make healthy food selections to nourish your body and mind, and prepare your body to conquer stress and disease.
3. Remove yourself from toxic situations both at work and at home. If a person is physically or verbally abusive toward you, even if you love the person, give yourself permission to set limits and depart from the situation.
4. Take short vacations to regroup throughout the year and designate time for a longer vacation during the year.
5. Avoid patterns of volatile arguments from persons who are preoccupied with their own emotions and peace, and not yours.
6. Exercise daily. Even a short walk around the block or in nature, lifting weights, or stretching can help build balance and strength.
7. Have faith that you are not alone in this world or universe. Explore spirituality and your belief in God.
8. Understand that your beauty is both inward and outward. If you are content with a new hairstyle or outfit and others do not like your outfit or hairstyle, own what you like and love it. Consciously decide to just be you.
9. Leave work on time.
10. Let no one define your worth both at work or home.

While this is by no means an exhaustive list of ways to simplify one's life, it is a start. The tips are free and most can be completed with minimal to no monetary amounts. Remember, taking a vacation at home with time off from work can be gratifying. Or taking a day off to explore the beach or experiment with new hairstyles or clothing or obtaining a massage can be relaxing. The key is to find something that is relaxing and people who bring "life to your life" through positivity and genuine care that is unconditional.

Here Is an Idea: Just Go to the Workplace to Work

If healthcare environments are to be therapeutic and intellectually stimulating with innovation being the ultimate goal for the healthcare team's achievement of individual patients' optimal wellness, workplace health must be prioritized. When workplace environments in healthcare are driven by therapeutics, quiet, respect, peace, and the subjective and objective focus on states of health, both patients and employees can thrive. The loneliness, isolation, and vulnerability experienced by patients, must not be overshadowed by the trust, expertise, and genuine care for humanity that healthcare workers offer patients as workers within healthcare settings.

The trivialness of The Hollow with senseless acts of targeted bullying is not appropriate to environments cultivating health and wellness. Hence The Hollow is not conducive to the workplace, let alone those, particularly those persons caring for vulnerable populations diagnosed with physical and mental illness. The practical approach to protection from The Hollow is to simply establish workplace policies whereby bullying is not tolerated. Demonstrations of uncivil conduct toward others is viewed as unprofessional and grounds for a progressive plan of action up to and including termination.

Why Do I Suffer at Work?

Therapeutic work with persons who experience workplace incivility can be disheartening. Hearing their pain and the injustices they have experienced on a frequent basis, often at no fault of their own, warrants organizational investigation, support, and resolution. It is also important for organizations to understand that unhealthy workplaces are an international phenomenon. The United Nations, in a global survey, found that one in five employees (23%) have been harassed and or experienced violence in the workplace that was sexual, psychological, or physical in nature. Of concern, according to the United Nations' International Labour Organization (2022) is the lack of disclosure by affected persons. With more women (60.7%) than men (50.1%), reporting their workplace incivility experiences because of their desire to protect their reputation, leaving persons who have been abusive to them in the workplace environment, or thinking disclosure to be a waste of their time, there is underreporting of uncivil conduct.

No matter the color of persons skin, the language they speak, the religion(s) they choose to practice, or the culture of which they originate, discrimination is illogical and unsettling and propagates disunity. Unity and healing must be the focus in order to disarm The Hollow and disempower bullies. In order for this to happen in the workplace, policies must be put in place that do not tolerate the wrongful treatment of employees by employees and employees with clients. Respect, not in word alone but indeed and action and without contingency plans, is what communicates care.

Workplace Norms

The Hollow challenges workplace norms that perpetuate self-destruction and the destruction of others. The nurturing workplace is one that seeks to resolve conflict, bring forth solutions, and sustain healthy work environments. Workplace norms that set forth the expectation of gratitude, supporting one another, and the importance of truth-telling are not representative of an idealistic Utopia but can easily be made a reality. Examples of workplace norms include the following:

- Zero tolerance for defamation of character in writing or orally.
- Affected parties and non-affected parties of bullying are provided the opportunity to confidentially express their experiences working within a toxic work environment.
- Ambiguous platitudes of others' character are thoroughly investigated to substantiate accuracy.
- Patterns of possible discrimination are investigated thoroughly by the organization.
- Annually, classes are provided on bullying prevention and reporting of toxic workplace experiences at identified system levels; employees to managers to directors to administrators and administrative teams and board members are treated as equal occurrences by the organizations, because all employees and persons that work, receive care, or interface with the organization have value.
- Progressive disciplinary action will be taken against repeat offenders and will include termination if no change in behaviors or actions occurs.
- Policies are reviewed annually to determine if an update is required for continual support and protection of all employees against The Hollow.

By upholding workplace norms, employees and employers have a contractual dialogue and agreement to maintain healthy workplace environments.

Who Says "No" Is Such a Bad Word in the Workplace?

The word "no" can be the most difficult words to say in the workplace, especially for the workaholic and dedicated employee. However, setting of limits creates work-life balance and job satisfaction. This same ability to set limits by saying "no" to workaholism and over dedication to the workplace for one's health and well-being must be applied to saying "no" to behaviors and actions representative of The Hollow in the workplace.

The word "no" brings clarity and focus as well as a well-defined understanding that the preservation of one's mental and physical health is a priority. It is the clear communication from the individual needing to say "no" that they value their own peace and will not allow anyone to disrupt their peace using disrespectful or dishonest approaches in the work environment. Individuals experiencing The Hollow in the workplace must make the conscious decision to never place their health in the hands of another person who has blatantly disrespected them.

Common Sense

Common sense is the basic sensibility applied in the recognition that a wrong or a right has occurred. The hierarchy of that which is civil and representative of truth is the absence of common sense necessity and a humane courtesy to be respectful. Having a mindset of unity is the only way to bring conflict resolution to a bullying situation.

Individuals who observe a gap of unification of employees within their organization would do well for themselves and their fellow employees to acknowledge the existence of dysfunction. The acknowledgment of the existence of The Hollow can help employees to assist their organization in changing the culture. A healthy work culture incorporates respect and unity of employees despite their differences.

And So, I Recall: Learning from the Past

If your organizational culture was affected by The Hollow in the past, this does not mean that there cannot be a reoccurrence of workplace bullying. A reoccurrence of bullying is always one employee hire away of a person with anger, integrity, manipulation, insecurity, or prior bullying issues. Hence, it is important that managers learn to ask questions and explore work history indicative of bullying behaviors. For example, a hiring manager could inquire about team-building skills and approaches to resolutions of conflict in the workplace and create scenarios whereby in writing, future employees must address a challenging fellow employee or client. Also, include a scenario, whereby the employee is a witness to an actual incident of bullying in the workplace, and ask the employee to explain how they would react and why they chose to react the way they did.

Pre-employment Screening: Two Scenario Examples:

Scenario 1: Addressing a Challenging Patient
The nurse enters the hospital room of a patient the nurse has been providing care to for the last 8 h of a 12-h shift. The nurse who answered the patient's call bell asks, "How may I help you." The patient shares, "I've decided that I want to change hospitals. I am not pleased with my care you provided me today. You are not a very good nurse, and you have a horrible bedside manner. I have already notified Patient Relations and your Manager. I am calling to ask you to pack my belongings and complete my discharge. I am ready to go!"

Answer the following questions:

1. What would be your first response?
2. Do you need to contact anyone?

3. Is there a need for follow-up with patient relations and the manager?
4. What education, if any, is necessary for the patient?
5. What education, if any, is necessary for you?
6. What is your greatest fear or concern after this verbal interaction with your patient?
7. Have you ever experienced a situation similar to the scenario? If yes, how did you handle it?
8. Is it common for patients to have complaints?
9. What is your motto in the care of patients that have shared that they are not pleased with their healthcare?
10. What would be your tone of voice, physical approach, proximity, and comfort level in engaging this patient in determining what could be done differently to ensure continuity of care and that they complete their healthcare treatment?

Scenario 2: Observing an Employee Being Bullied
At 7:45 p.m., you have just completed your 12-h day to evening shift and begin walking toward the fifth level of the garage where you parked earlier. As you walk toward your car, you hear arguing, and someone whispering, "If you tell anyone, I will deny it and you'll look like the fool. They will believe me over you any day." Standing quietly behind a truck in a darkened area of the garage, you observe that it is the female assistant nurse manager and a male nurse from your unit. You hear the male nurse say, "I am back with my wife and our child. I am ending this relationship that should have never begun in the first place. I made a mistake. My wife forgives me and I am moving on."

The female assist nurse manager slaps the male nurse on his left cheek and begins to walk away stating, "I will get you fired. If I have to lie about your character, I will get you fired."

Answer the following questions:

1. What would you do?
2. Should you make your presence known to your two co-workers in the garage?
3. Is it necessary to approach either party to explain what you heard them discuss?
4. Would you disclose what you heard to another employee you work with?
5. Whom should the information you heard be shared with within the organization?
6. Is employee confidentiality important in this situation?
7. What is your role here, if any?
8. Who are you advocating for in this situation?
9. What type of situation is this?
10. Have you ever participated within or observed workplace bullying before? If yes, what was the outcome?

Hiring managers should review the scenario and responses with the future employee to provide an opportunity for him or her to explain their thought processes in answering the questions and also to determine how they interpreted the scenario itself. Include their feedback and your discussion with the future employee as part of their scenario write-up. The latter is an opportunity to provide future hires with insight on the importance of healthy workplace environments. With regard to whether the individual is hired or not, an opportunity to promote healthy workplace ideals has been provided.

References

Cook-Campbell, A. (2023). How to have a good work-life balance. *Betterup*. https://www.betterup.com/blog/how-to-have-good-work-life-balance#what-does-work-life-balance-mean?

el Batawi, M. A. (1984). Work-related diseases. A new program of the World Health Organization. *Scandinavian Journal of Work Environmental Health, 10*(6 Spec No), 341–346. doi:https://doi.org/10.5271/sjweh.2309

Gragnano, A., Simbula, S., & Miglioretti, M. (2020). Work-life balance: Weighing the importance of work-family and work-health balance. *International Journal of Environmental Research & Public Health, 17*(3), 907. https://doi.org/10.3390/ijerph17030907

Kivimäki, M., Jokela, M., Nyberg, S. T., Singh-Manoux, A., Fransson, E. I., Alfredsson, L., Bjorner, J. B., Borritz, M., Burr, H., Casini, A., Clays, E., De Bacquer, D., Dragano, N., Erbel, R., Geuskens, G. A., Hamer, M., Hooftman, W. E., Houtman, I. L., Jöckel, K. H., Kittel, F., Knutsson, A., Koskenvuo, M., Lunau, T., Madsen, I. E., Nielsen, M. L., Nordin, M., Oksanen, T., Pejtersen, J. H., Pentti, J., Rugulies, R., Salo, P., Shipley, M. J., Siegrist, J., Steptoe, A., Suominen, S. B., Theorell, T., Vahtera, J., Westerholm, P. J., Westerlund, H., O'Reilly, D., Kumari, M., Batty, G. D., Ferrie, J. E., & Virtanen, M. (2015). IPD-work consortium. Long working hours and risk of coronary heart disease and stroke: A systematic review and meta-analysis of published and unpublished data for 603,838 individuals. *Lancet, 386*(10005), 1739–1746. https://doi.org/10.1016/S0140-6736(15)60295-1

United Nations. (2022, December 5). More than 1 in 5 worldwide suffering from violence at work: ILO. United Nations International Labour Organization. https://news.un.org/en/story/2022/12/1131272

Virtanen, M., Ferrie, J. E., Singh-Manoux, A., Shipley, M. J., Stansfeld, S. A., Marmot, M. G., Ahola, K., Vahtera, J., & Kivimäki, M. (2011). Long working hours and symptoms of anxiety and depression: A 5-year follow-up of the Whitehall II study. *Psychological Medicine, 41*(12), 2485–2494. https://doi.org/10.1017/S0033291711000171

A Coverage of Eyes and Ears

10

Learning Objectives

1. Consider the implications of choosing not to advocate for a person heard and or observed being bullied.
2. Explain how ignoring bullying in the workplace impacts not only the affected person but the observer as well.

Eyes and Ears

The **eyes and ears** reveal a multitude of sins. For persons targeted by bullies in the workplace and experiencing The Hollow, the hope for a witness who observed and or heard the bully or bullies being offensive is important to the substantiation of their complaint. However, when persons observing and hearing incidences of workplace bullying choose to be silent, the toxicity of the workplace remains. Over longer periods of time in workplaces, the silence of standby observers and hearers serves to empower the bullies so that bullying persists and more targets are identified.

Secondary Trauma

For nurses experiencing The Hollow in the context of workplace bullying, they can feel isolated, helpless, and hopeless. Interestingly, for nurses or other persons observing and hearing workplace bullying, whether they choose to report the bullying or do not, secondary trauma can occur. **Secondary trauma** can occur when a person is exposed to another person who is involved in a traumatizing event such as workplace bullying (e.g., yelling, harassment, belittlement, lying, mobbing, social exclusion, etc.).

Jiao et al. (2023) noted that persons who were bullied over long periods of time were more likely to report post-traumatic stress disorder, helplessness, anger, sleep disruption, silence, depression, powerlessness, and anger. Ongoing exposure led to digestive problems, stress, decreased immunity, high blood pressure, and headaches.

Summary

Observers and hearers of bullying can help to end the bully or bullies' negative behavior and actions by acknowledging what they saw and reporting the negative behavior to their manager, director, and Human Resources Department. It is important that it be emphasized within healthcare organizations experiencing bullying, particularly bullying that is nurse-to-nurse, that a zero tolerance for bullying being adopted to maintain a healthy workplace environment (ANA, 2015; Knight et al., 2024) is necessary for the health and well-being of employees. Policies adhering to zero tolerance should be developed and require employee signature sign off annually to hold perpetrators accountable. Organizations that ignore bullying and that condone employees who ignore bullying are placing the lives of nurses at risk and, ultimately, endangering the lives of patients treated by nurses who are the walking wounded victims of The Hollow.

References

American Nurses Association. (2015). *Incivility, bullying, and workplace violence*. ANA position statement. https://www.nursingworld.org/practice-policy/nursing-excellence/official-position-statements/id/incivility-bullying-and-workplace-violence/

Jiao, R., Li, J., Cheng, N., Liu, X., & Tan, Y. (2023). The mediating role of coping styles between nurses' workplace bullying and professional quality of life. *BMC Nursing, 22*(1), 1–10. https://doi-org.acu.idm.oclc.org/10.1186/s12912-023-01624-y

Knight, K. E., Ellis, C., Miller, T., Neu, J., & Helfrich, L. (2024). Does where you work and what you do matter? Testing the role of organizational context and job type for future study of occupation-based secondary trauma intervention development. *Journal of Interpersonal Violence, 39*(7–8), 1623–1648. https://doi-org.acu.idm.oclc.org/10.1177/08862605231211927

Is a State of Calm Achievable? 11

Learning Objectives

1. Discuss how a state of calm can be maintained during The Hollow experience.
2. Discuss how a state of calm can be met and sustained post The Hollow experience.

A History of Abuse

In 1909, an article written in The New York Times newspaper revealed how head nurses (now referred to as nurse managers) harassed and insulted their staff nurses (The New York Times, 1909). Historically, nurses have endured bullying within the workplace for years. These unhealthy behaviors negatively affect nurses. Without the opportunity for calm and moments of peace and tranquility, nurses affected by bullying can have difficulty functioning within their positions as licensed professionals serving the public.

Calm

Calm is a state of peace and tranquility. To become calm is to be relaxed, not agitated or restless. During the experience of bullying, it is imperative that persons affected maintain a state of calm when interfacing with the bully or bullies. A state of calm may be subjectively protective in the maintenance of mental and physical health.

When calm, the person within the bullying situation being bullied can process what is occurring, identify the perpetrator's(s') weaknesses and strengths, and engage in addressing the end of the bullying itself. Calm brings a sense of control. Calm will end the bullying as it brings clarity and a divine wisdom to a situation that is otherwise out of control.

Achievable

When something is **achievable**, it is soon to be completed. Although peace and calm seem unachievable in the midst of The Hollow, both can be accomplished. For persons affected by The Hollow, with counseling and the support of family and friends, the reestablishment of a work-life balance can be achieved. While immediate forgiveness can be difficult, releasing oneself from the perceived power of the bully or bullies comes when the affected person recognizes their personal value and worth as priceless and perseveration on a bully or bullies in their life, a waste of their time. Calm will be sustained post bullying when affected persons use the experience to empower themselves and others as they educate about bullying prevention and consequences.

Ultimately, change will occur, but it may or may not be in the workplace the bullying occurred but in the person affected themselves. Persons affected by The Hollow never maneuver nor experience their daily interactions inside and outside of the workplace the same. They are more aware of other's dysfunction, and their own physiological and psychological responses to potential displays of bullying.

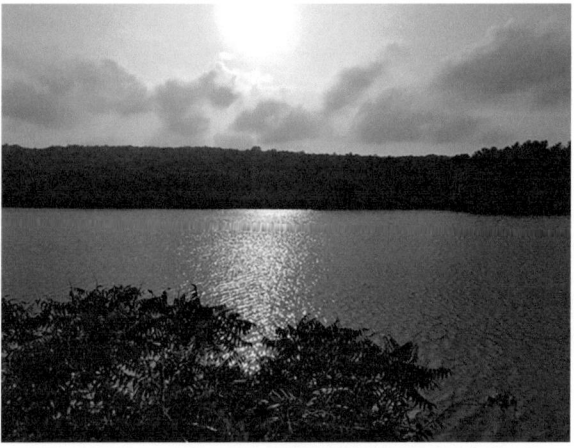

Calm

Activity

The Use of Mindfulness in Healing from The Hollow

Williams and Penman (2011) describe mindfulness as being simple and worthwhile because mindfulness exercises can prevent spiraling periods of sadness accompanied by prolonged periods of exhaustion and unhappiness—clinical depression, stress, and anxiety.

With the business of daily lives, a 1-min mindful meditation can provide a brief relief from unplanned disruptions that can temporarily exhaust and cause feelings of stress. Here are three 1-min mediations below.

One-Minute Meditation

Number 1. Basic Start of the Day

1. Standing upright, take a deep breath, and raise both arms as if stretching to touch the ceiling (or sky if outdoors).
2. Close your eyes. As you close your eyes, take a deep breath.
3. The breath you take is needed to sustain life. Your life.
4. Listen to your breath. Feel your breath. Become aware of your own breathing and how it sounds.
5. Place you left and right hands on your chest. Slow your breathing down. Be aware of the rise and fall of your chest.
6. Stretch your hands toward the ceiling (or sky if outdoors). Reach as if attempting to touch the ceiling (or sky). Lower your hands and relax.
7. Be thankful for the moment and the pause you took to care for yourself.
8. Resume your day.

One-Minute Meditation

Number 2. Thankful Breath

1. Allow for privacy and quiet.
2. Sit in a chair.
3. Ground yourself. Feet flat on the floor with shoes removed. Lower back against the chair. Sit erect.
4. Close your eyes.
5. Take a deep breath. Place your hands on your abdomen. Pull in your abdomen inward as you take a deep breath. Hold the breath and count to three--- 1---2---3.
6. Slowly release the breath.
7. At the end of the breath quietly state the word "Thankful."
8. Repeat this exercise three times.
9. Our breath honors our very existence. Our breath represents life. Our verbalization of the word "Thankful" is a reminder to appreciate our own existence.
10. When we honor our existence, we can begin to appreciate not only ourselves but also our fellow human beings (e.g., co-workers) who exist and have breath as we do.

One-Minute Meditation

Number 3. Calming Break with Visualization

1. Obtain a pen or pencil with one blank piece of paper.
2. Place the writing utensil and blank piece of paper on a desk or table.
3. Sit in front of the desk or table.
4. Sit erect.
5. Feet grounded: shoes on or off.
6. Close your eyes.
7. Count to six----1---2---3---4---5---6.
8. Open your eyes.
9. Fix your eyes on the writing utensil and blank piece of paper.
10. Close your eyes.
11. Think of a quiet place that you would like to visit. The place could be a beach, your home, a favorite chair, or a favorite restaurant eating a tasty meal.
12. Mentally draw the picture using your imagination where you would like to visit.
13. Open your eyes and write down the place you visited and how it made you feel.
14. As you resume your day, select a date on your calendar to visit the place you selected.
15. Remember to take time to create mini vacations to rest, renew, and refresh.

Counseling

When a person experiences workplace bullying, they may feel anxious, paranoid, betrayed, fearful, sad, lonely, isolated, and depressed. Episodes of tearfulness are not out of the ordinary. Unfortunately, the feelings associated with the workplace-based bullying are not solely manifested at work. Affected persons bring these feelings home and marriages and relationships with family members and friends are impacted as well. Hence, it is imperative that persons affected by The Hollow receive counseling.

By securing the services of a professional counselor or therapist, affected persons are providing themselves the opportunity to process their feelings and the emotional pain and turmoil they felt while being bullied within a safe and confidential setting. The processing of these varied emotions is necessary to deter the development of psychiatric disorders such as posttraumatic stress disorder, anxiety disorders, panic disorders, eating disorders, obsessive compulsive disorders, or depressive disorders (Halter Jordan, 2022).

References

Halter Jordan, M. (2022). *Varcarolis' foundations of psychiatric-mental health nursing: A clinical approach* (9th ed.). Elsevier.

The New York Times. (1909, August 22). In Castronovo, M. A., Pullizzi, A., & Evans, S. (2016). Nurse bullying: A review and a proposed solution. *Nursing Outlook, 64*(3), 208–214. https://doi.org/10.1016/j.outlook.2015.11.008

Williams, M., & Penman, D. (2011). *Mindfulness: An eight-week plan for finding peace in a frantic world*. Rodale.

Arise and Journey More

12

Learning Objectives

1. Consider the next steps of the nurse affected by bullying.
2. Discuss if a change in workplace environment resolves the problem of The Hollow.
3. Recognize if the nurse affected by workplace bullying decides to remain at the workplace at which the bullying occurred that he or she will require emotional support and allowance for personal growth and empowerment in order to heal.

Arise

Change is necessary for progress to occur. With workplace bullying, if the culture is allowed to remain unchanged, bullying with arise again. Hence, it is imperative that organizations **arise** or bring into existence a culture of zero tolerance (ANA, 2015) for bullying and embrace and support nurses who have experienced bullying within these organizations' four walls.

Journey More

For nurses who experience the hollow, the opportunity to **journey more** (work in a healthy workplace) may not come in the absence of organizational recognition that they have a bullying problem. In order to create healthy workplaces, the illnesses of sick workplaces must be identified and resolved. The latter meaning, bullies must be held accountable, and the mental health (counseling) needs of both the bullies and affected nurses prioritized. If bullies continue to exhibit negative behaviors, termination post-mental health (counseling) treatment should be an option. Healthy workplaces are of the upmost importance for nurses, particularly because nurses have the very serious responsibility of providing healthcare to the public (Cleary et al., 2010; Ganz et al., 2015; Salmeron & Christian, 2016; Wilson, 2016). A bullied nurse is a psychologically and physiologically impaired nurse.

Emotional Support

Emotional support involves the skill of silently listening to the sorrows or burdens of another. Vaclavikova et al. (2022) conducted a scoping review of 573 articles on mobbing. A review of the articles that included Scopus, Ovid Nursing, Taylor and Francis, and EBSCOhost yielded a total of 23 articles that were reviewed on the topic of mobbing occurring with nurses in the workplace. Mobbing is a type of workplace bullying that involves behaviors such as constant criticism, ignoring, discrediting, humiliation, gossiping, and isolation (Efe & Ayaz, 2010; Leymann, 1996; Suárez García, 2021) as a means to psychologically exhaust the affected person with the goal of facilitating the person's departure from the workplace. Nurses impacted by mobbing require **emotional support** due to their having experienced intentionally planned abusive behaviors within their work environment.

Vaclavikova et al. (2022), after completing a scoping review of the literature, identified the following mobbing prevention interventions that were effective in the workplace: clear rules and sanctions (Kim & Sim, 2021), adequate awareness (Castronovo et al., 2016; Pai & Lee, 2011; Stagg et al., 2013), cooperative team leadership (Bortoluzzi et al., 2014; Johnson, 2015; Ruíz-González et al., 2020), and good communication skills (Asi Karakaş & Okanli, 2015; Keller et al., 2016). From an organizational perspective, mobbing is a serious issue because it can lead to nursing turnover and creates an environment whereby uncivil conduct is allowed to proliferate at the expense of the mental health of nurses. Hence it is imperative that all staff working within healthcare organizations be provided training on mobbing behaviors, how to identify them, skills to effectively intervene when a colleague is experiencing bullying via mobbing, and how to report persons perpetuating mobbing behaviors against the affected person(s). In the case of mobbing, having knowledge is having the power to prevent this bullying behavior.

Personal Growth

Personal growth can occur after a person experiences bullying within the workplace.
Personal growth occurs when a person seeks to understand themselves and the people in their lives, finds meaning in their relationships and careers, and has found personal fulfillment in their spiritual life. Personal growth occurs when an individual decides that being stagnant in life is not living life to the fullest.

Roberts Morgan et al. (2019) found in their research using the tool they developed entitled Reflected Best Self Exercise (RBSE) in 2005, that when people receive positive feedback about their contributions and strengths, they become more emotionally healthy. Emotionally healthy people tend to have good relationships with their colleagues, family, and friends and are resourceful and build personal agency. Presumptively, these are people, who in the workplace environment will have an increase in job satisfaction.

Roberts Morgan et al. (2019) identified five practices that can enhance personal growth through the development of your *best self*. These five practices are:

1. Notice positive feedback
2. Ask questions
3. Study your successes
4. Practice enacting your best self
5. Pay it forward

When an individual makes a point to listen to the positive feedback of others and not just focus on the negative comments of a few people, they can become their best self. By asking questions to learn more and demonstrate a genuine interest in the lives and work of others, a person can become their best self. Taking the time to reflect on one's own successes in their professional and personal life makes one thankful. Each day, making the decision to begin and end your day by recognizing your contributions not only within the work environment but at church or perhaps a place that you do volunteer work in the community, makes your workplace small and your personal world larger. Hence, you have accomplishments outside of the workplace and do not define yourself solely by your job. Lastly, always remember the importance of honoring the accomplishments of others. Everyone has the potential to do great work at work and beyond!

Empowerment

Persons experiencing **empowerment** are autonomous and feel in control of their lives despite life stressors and complexities. The obtainment of empowerment during and after having experienced bullying should be the healthy goal of all impacted by The Hollow. The attainment of empowerment involves persons affected by The Hollow having insight into their situation and being able to clearly identify situations whereby the negative behaviors were encountered, as well as their participation in the toleration of the acts of bullying in absence of reporting the incidences to others. Persons who feel empowered are not victims but victors and are able to view negative behaviors directed at them as not being representative of whom they personally or professionally nor representative of the value or the talent and gifts they bring to the workplace.

References

American Nurses Association. (2015). *Incivility, bullying, and workplace violence*. ANA position statement. https://www.nursingworld.org/practice-policy/nursing-excellence/official-position-statements/id/incivility-bullying-and-workplace-violence/

Asi Karakaş, S., & Okanli, A. E. (2015). The effect of assertiveness training on the mobbing that nurses experience. *Workplace Health & Safety, 63*(10), 446–451. https://doi.org/10.1177/2165079915591708

Bortoluzzi, G., Caporale, L., & Palese, A. (2014). Does participative leadership reduce the onset of mobbing risk among nurse working teams? *Journal of Nursing Management, 22*(5), 643–652. https://doi.org/10.1111/jonm.12042

Castronovo, M. A., Pullizzi, A., & Evans, S. (2016). Nurse bullying: A review and a proposed solution. *Nursing Outlook, 64*(3), 208–214. https://doi.org/10.1016/j.outlook.2015.11.008

Cleary, M., Hunt, G. E., & Horsfall, J. (2010). Identifying and addressing bullying in nursing. *Issues in Mental Health Nursing, 31*(5), 331–335. https://doi.org/10.3109/01612840903308531

Efe, S. Y., & Ayaz, S. (2010). Mobbing against nurses in the workplace in Turkey. *International Nursing Review, 57*(3), 328–334. https://doi.org/10.1111/j.1466-7657.2010.00815.x

Ganz, F. D., Levy, H., Khalaila, R., Arad, D., Bennaroch, K., Kolpak, O., Drori, Y., Benbinishty, J., & Raanan, O. (2015). Bullying and its prevention among intensive care nurses. *Journal of Nursing Scholarship, 47*(6), 505–511. https://doi.org/10.1111/jnu.12167

Johnson, S. L. (2015). Workplace bullying prevention: A critical discourse analysis. *Journal of Advanced Nursing, 71*(10), 2384–2392. https://doi.org/10.1111/jan.12694

Keller, R., Budin, W. C., & Allie, T. (2016). A task force to address bullying. *AJN The American Journal of Nursing, 116*(2), 52–58. https://doi.org/10.1097/01.NAJ.0000480497.63846.d0

Kim, H. S., & Sim, I. O. (2021). The experience of clinical nurses after Korea's enactment of workplace anti-bullying legislation: A phenomenological study. *International Journal of Environmental Research and Public Health, 18*(11), 5711. https://doi.org/10.3390/ijerph18115711

Leymann, H. (1996). The content and development of mobbing at work. *European Journal of Work and Organizational Psychology, 5*(2), 165–184. https://doi.org/10.1080/13594329608414853

Pai, H. C., & Lee, S. (2011). Risk factors for workplace violence in clinical registered nurses in Taiwan. *Journal of Clinical Nursing, 20*(9–10), 1405–1412. https://doi.org/10.1111/j.1365-2702.2010.03650.x

Roberts Morgan, L., Heaphy, E., & Caza, B. (2019, May 14). Personal Growth and Transformation: To become your best self, study your successes. *Harvard Business Review*. https://hbr.org/2019/05/to-become-your-best-self-study-your-successes.

Ruíz-González, K. J., Pacheco-Pérez, L. A., García-Bencomo, M. I., Diez, M. G., & Guevara-Valtier, M. C. (2020). Mobbing perception among intensive care unit nurses. *Enfermería Intensiva (English ed.), 31*(3), 113–119. https://doi.org/10.1016/j.enfie.2019.03.007

Salmeron, P. A., & Christian, B. J. (2016). Evaluation of an educational program to improve school nursing staff perceptions of bullying in Pinellas County, Florida. *Pediatric Nursing, 42*(6), 283–292.

Stagg, S. J., Sheridan, D. J., Jones, R. A., & Speroni, K. G. (2013). Workplace bullying: The effectiveness of a workplace program. *Workplace Health & Safety, 61*(8), 333–338. https://doi.org/10.1177/216507991306100803

Suárez García, S. (2021). El mobbing en el sector turístico: ¿realidad o ficción? [Mobbing in the tourism sector: Fact or fiction?]. *Trascender, contabilidad y gestión, 6*(18), 41–52. https://doi.org/10.36791/tcg.v0i18.127

Vaclavikova, K., Soukalova, K., Kopecky, M., & Molnarova, L. (2022). Preventing mobbing of nurses: A scoping review. *Central European Journal of Nursing & Midwifery, 14*(3), 956–964. https://cejnm.osu.cz/artkey/cjn-202303-0002_preventing-mobbing-of-nurses-a-scoping-review.php?back=%2Fsearch.php%3Fquery%3DNursing%2Bnow%2Bin%253Aauth%2Bname%2Bkey%2Babstr%26sfrom%3D30%26spage%3D30

Wilson, J. L. (2016). An exploration of bullying behaviors in nursing: A review of the literature. *British Journal of Nursing, 25*(6), 303–306. https://doi.org/10.12968/bjon.2016.25.6.303

Conclusion: The Gratitude Effect Booklet

Nurses experience The Hollow question why they are being bullied. Additionally, these nurses seek to understand outside of themselves, their purpose after the trauma of bullying, and how they can move forward past the experience. The Gratitude Booklet, written by Lance Bane explores the importance of gratitude in moving beyond past hurt.

Lance Bane Lance's greatest joys are his relationship with King Jesus, his wife, Darlene, his three kids, and his grandkids. Lance views the world through the lens of hope and believes that each problem is an opportunity to grow, learn, and help. Mark Twain once said, "The two most important days in your life are the day you are born, and the day you find out why." He hopes that, through a relationship with Jesus Christ, you will discover God's love and share that love with the world.

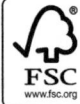

MIX
Papier aus verantwortungsvollen Quellen
Paper from responsible sources
FSC® C105338

If you have any concerns about our products,
you can contact us on
ProductSafety@springernature.com

In case Publisher is established outside the EU,
the EU authorized representative is:
Springer Nature Customer Service Center GmbH
Europaplatz 3, 69115 Heidelberg, Germany

Printed by Libri Plureos GmbH
in Hamburg, Germany